# my Gut

## IBS, SIBO and other digestive issues

### ADA J. PETERS

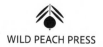

WILD PEACH PRESS

# DISCLAIMER

This book contains content relating to physical and/or mental health and has been written for informational and educational purposes only. The author acknowledges that she is not a professional healthcare provider. Her work is based on extensive research and personal experience. Every effort has been made to ensure that the information contained in this book is accurate.

The ideas, procedures and suggestions expressed in this book are not intended as a substitute for advice from a licensed healthcare provider, such as your doctor. All health matters require medical supervision. If you think the information in this book may be of value to you, consult your doctor to determine if the suggestions and recommendations made in this book can be incorporated into your treatment.

The author and publisher shall not be liable for any injury, damage or loss allegedly arising from any information or suggestions in this book. The author is not liable for the content of third parties to which she refers for further information, be they persons, organizations, or websites. The reader should also be aware that internet sites listed in this work may become inaccessible over time. This book was written and published independently and with no third-party sponsorship, affiliation, or endorsement.

Published by Wild Peach Press Pty Ltd

www.wildpeachpress.com

First edition

ISBN (Paperback):    978-0-6456786-0-4


Front cover: Textile artwork by Kate Theobald

To all those who are brave enough to embark on the journey to develop a more intimate relationship with their body and soul.

# CONTENTS

# INTRODUCTION

Unfortunately, millions of people around the world suffer from gastro-intestinal symptoms such as constipation, diarrhea, bloating and pain, which are often accompanied by weight concerns, food intolerances, skin problems and mental health issues. If you are among them, you may know all too well how frustrating it is to find an answer to these health problems. All the more reason to congratulate you for setting out on the quest to find out more about conditions like Irritable Bowel Syndrome (IBS) and Small Intestinal Bacterial Overgrowth (SIBO). There are no easy answers on this journey, because there is no one-size-fits-all solution to overcome these disorders. Our bodies, our life circumstances and the causes are too different for that.

Each patient usually receives an individual treatment that takes these conditions into account, which is often enough refined through many trials and errors. To minimize this process this book presents the latest scientific findings, complemented by my personal experience, to answer the most important questions that may arise. This information allows you to make informed choices.

During my own health journey, I realized that focusing on the physical body is only half of the story – the other half is the influence of the intestinal tract on mental and emotional wellbeing, or vice versa. Depression, mood swings and a foggy brain often originate in a compromised digestive system. Additional stress - whether physical or psychological – is another reason recovery may be hindered. In this book you will find a wealth of information on these topics that will help you to deal with mental health problems and the various types of stress.

By gaining a deeper understanding of IBS, SIBO and related conditions, you can apply strategies to take back control of your health. When you know where compromised gut health comes from, how to alleviate symptoms and make simple lifestyle changes, you can contribute to a lasting improvement in health. Diet is usually the first approach to manage IBS and SIBO. I can still remember how stressful it was not to know what to eat. I felt vulnerable and confused. Everything I thought was healthy food suddenly no longer worked for me. To give you a better start, I am going to cover the topic of food in more detail.

Whether you are at the beginning or in the middle of your journey to recovery, don't be too hard on yourself. There is no point in blaming the bacteria in your intestines or yourself. It is neither a competition nor a fight to overcome this situation, but rather an ongoing process of detaching oneself from the circumstances that contributed to the development of these conditions. Accepting that you are not in complete control of the causes can be a first step towards healing. Be compassionate and gentle with yourself as you develop a new relationship with your body. This doesn't mean you should bury your head in the sand, but rather, learn to listen and nourish yourself as best you can. Take one step at a time and make changes towards a healthier and more sustainable lifestyle.

I wish you all the best of health.
Ada

# MY STORY

My intestinal problems started when I was as a young child in Germany. It was the 1960s, and the medical world and society had not yet developed the extensive knowledge of intestinal health that we have today. The internet was still decades away, and people had to rely solely on a doctor's medical wisdom. At the time, I was as thin as a stick and could not gain weight. When I was sixteen years old, I thought it was normal to pass stools only once a week. My first endoscopy showed the onset of ulcerative colitis, which is an inflammatory bowel disease. The gastroenterologist did not recommend any particular treatment, food, or lifestyle change. I thought "It can't be that bad" and so I went on with my life. Depression hit me in my mid-twenties, and a foggy brain was familiar to me.

In the 1980s, a friend suggested I see a naturopath who discovered that I had certain bacteria missing from my stool. At that time it felt a little strange, someone looking at my poop and making a treatment plan based on what they found. Being a student, I was not able to afford any further consultations with this naturopath. I got used to my symptoms and was in denial that there was anything wrong with me. Suddenly, in my thirties, I gained a lot of weight. The change was quite shocking, as I no longer recognized myself in the mirror. In addition, I felt endlessly tired. A further medical consultation lead to the advice that I should get a high-fiber supplement from the chemist or take some laxatives. Both made me feel worse.

After moving to Australia, I became pregnant with twin boys. During the pregnancy I developed type 2 diabetes. This prompted me to follow a diet that was almost free of sugar, carbohydrates, and processed foods. I simply ate lots of fresh salads, vegetables and some meat. I felt fantastic for the first time in my life! Thankfully, the diabetes disappeared after the birth of my boys, but things changed rapidly in another direction. Since I was always hungry while nursing, I felt I could eat a whole truckload at each meal. To satisfy my needs, my diet changed to pasta, couscous, and other carbohydrates. Suddenly, I was permanently bloated. Any possible damage from giving birth was ruled out and I was tested for celiac disease; the result came back negative.

I was so busy with the babies that I could not continue to take care of my health. I pushed all signs of illness out of my consciousness, although there were many hints that something was wrong. Irregular bowel movements with stools that were hard to flush, fatigue (who would not be tired with twin babies?), a foggy brain, severe back pain and skin irritations were just some of them. I would tell myself there was nothing to worry about: "Doesn't everyone have health issues to some degree?" I guessed that I just needed sleep, the right face cream, to go to the gym, eat less, and avoid drinking milk.

One day, at the airport, a flight attendant looked at my belly and asked for a letter of consent from my doctor before I was allowed to board. She thought I was pregnant. I wasn't. I was, as usual, just bloated. This embarrassing incident prompted me to do some research for this condition. This time I was ready to find an answer to my problems. On my journey to better health I saw many doctors and specialists. They all looked at certain parts of my problem and gave me all sorts of recommendations: eat more avocados and steak, take more supplements, use a therapeutic face cream for rosacea, or don't worry so much as it was just my age. The worst statement I heard was, "Your problem is that you are too healthy". This comment was hard to take as I could barely stand upright at this point due to severe vertigo. It was incredibly frustrating, as I didn't know what else I could do or where to go. Researching on the internet made everything worse as the medical jargon overwhelmed me and I got lost in a mountain of details. I was wandering in the dark for many years and spent a vast amount of money on various diagnoses that were basically just hunches.

My doctor suggested I see a heart specialist to find out why I have vertigo and fatigue. This thoughtful man told me that I probably had a problem with my gut rather than my heart. Surprise! Shortly after this consultation, I was booked in for an endoscopy and a colonoscopy. The diagnosis was IBS, celiac disease – although I had previously tested negative to this disease – and the remission of ulcerative colitis. You can't imagine how relieved I was when I had real names for my health condition and could start to do more detailed research.

This led me to an elimination diet called the Specific Carbohydrate Diet, which is supposed to help with IBS. It is a strict diet. Until symptoms are under control, you should eat only a few different foods. Later, other foods are gradually introduced. However, it can take a long time before you have a reasonable selection of food in your diet again. It was hard, but I was fully committed to it. The first three months worked well for me as I did not experience bloating or have issues with bowel movements, but after a while, I wondered if I was on the right track. Although I took supplements and ate red meat, I was still deficient in iron and vitamin B12. Despite this, I continued with the diet. Unfortunately, I was slowly becoming my old, bloated self again. It was devastating. What had happened? Further research revealed information about SIBO. From there on, I had a vague feeling that I had more than just IBS. This "gut" feeling prompted me to do a test which revealed a methane dominant SIBO. With this new knowledge, I set out to find a doctor who was knowledgeable about IBS and SIBO. A new chapter of my health journey began. Still, it was a steep learning curve to figure out what had caused the conditions, and what approaches were best to help me. In this endeavor, researching and writing this book has helped me greatly. The purpose of this book is to share my knowledge with you in the hope that it will also pave the way to better health for you.

"Gut health is a state of physical and mental wellbeing
in the absence of gastrointestinal complaints
that require the consultation of a doctor,
in the absence of indications or risks of bowel disease,
and in the absence of confirmed bowel disease"

**World Health Organization**

# IRRITABLE BOWEL SYNDROME

IBS and SIBO are difficult to distinguish from each other, as their symptoms can be very similar. To complicate things further, these disorders might even occur simultaneously or stimulate each other. Depending on the individual health condition, a different treatment approach may be necessary. Many problems related to IBS are also part of SIBO or vice versa. Throughout this book, you will discover information that will be of benefit to both conditions.

IBS affects people all over the world regardless of gender, age and culture. Some people suffer only occasional symptoms, while others are severely impaired in their quality of life. IBS should not be confused with inflammatory bowel disease (IBD), a chronic inflammation of the gastrointestinal tract, while IBS is a functional disorder that can affect any part of the gastrointestinal system. It is unlikely that IBS causes inflammatory bowel disease, but the opposite may be true. People who are in remission with inflammatory bowel disease may experience symptoms that are actually caused by IBS. If this happens to you, please contact your doctor to check whether you have IBS as well so that you do not have to take unnecessary medication.

To assist diagnosis of IBS, the Rome IV criteria are usually considered by doctors as it covers a wide range of symptoms. These criteria were developed by scientists and experts to better understand this functional gastrointestinal disorder. According to these criteria IBS is classified into subtypes based on the consistency of the stool rather than the frequency of bowel movements. Types include IBS-C (constipation), IBS-D (diarrhea) and IBS-M (a mixture of lumpy and watery stool). Usually, a predisposition to IBS is required before it can develop. This may be genetic, or you may have been given too many antibiotics as a child. An acute gastroenteritis or stomach upset due to food poisoning or traveler's diarrhea strongly contribute to IBS. If the signs of these viral infections persist for weeks, there is an increased risk of developing post-infectious IBS (PI-IBS) that can become chronic. Other risk factors are a hypersensitivity of the gut, motility disorders, impaired transmission of pain signals from the gut to the brain, diet, and psychological influences such as chronic stress, anxiety and traumatic events from the past and present. For example, all forms of physical, emotional, and sexual abuse, in particular childhood sexual abuse.

Testing for IBS is limited. Patients with suspected IBS are usually given a complete blood count and other tests to rule out other diseases. For example, your doctor may request a blood test for celiac disease, a colonoscopy if polyps or inflammation, or a stool test to rule out parasites. Dr. Mark Pimentel, a leading expert in gut health and director of the Medically Associated Science and Technology (MAST) Program at Cedars-Sinai, and his team developed ibs-smart®, a test commonly used to diagnose IBS-D and IBS-M. It looks for specific antibodies (anti-CdtB and anti-vinculin) that are associated with food poisoning. It can distinguish between an inflammatory bowel disease and IBS without an invasive colonoscopy.

Most IBS symptoms are abdominal discomfort, bloating, and pain - usually on the left side of the abdomen - altered bowel movements such as diarrhea and constipation or an alternation of both, gas, visceral hypersensitivity, and unusual loud rumbling in the tummy. Non-colonic symptoms are back pain, fatigue, joint pain (fibromyalgia), bladder issues, pain during intercourse in woman, headaches, nausea or even occasional vomiting, chest pain, temperature during IBS flare ups, and anxiety. About 40–60% of patients with IBS admit that they suffer from depression, anxiety and/or somatization - the tendency to translate negative emotional thoughts and feelings into physical symptoms. It is still unknown whether these physiological symptoms are the cause or the effect of this disorder. IBS is more common in women than in men, in whom the symptoms are often less pronounced. Researchers found that responses to treatments may differ between the sexes, which should be taken into account by health professionals.

Many of these symptoms affect daily life to a greater or lesser extent. Those affected often feel embarrassed or worried when these come to light. For example, unpredictable diarrhea can trigger fears of not being able to get to the bathroom on time, being homebound, and even avoiding relationships because they feel ashamed of them. Diarrhea and constipation are the result of impaired gastrointestinal motility, meaning either too much or too little water is absorbed in the digestive process, resulting in faster or slower movement of bowel matter. A Johns Hopkins factsheet on IBS cites a study that found that, over a 24 hour interval, healthy participants had six to eight intestinal muscle contractions. Participants with IBS-C had almost none, and those with IBS-D had up to twenty-five contractions.

Sometimes diarrhea can mislead one, as it is actually a sign of constipation. When the lower part of the colon is clogged with hard stool, only liquid can flow around it, giving the impression of diarrhea - it is then called spurious diarrhea. If this condition is not properly diagnosed by your doctor through abdominal examination and/or an x-ray, it can become quite serious as an anti-diarrhea medication will make this condition worse.

> I went through a very stressful experience with my son, when he was a young child. He suffered from severe diarrhea, and to find out what was wrong with him, we consulted several doctors and a naturopath. They all examined him thoroughly and performed various tests. He was put on an elimination diet and was given nutritional supplements to combat the condition. These two years were difficult not only for him, but also for the whole family. The situation resolved itself when a pediatric gastroenterologist advised us to have an X-ray examination. My poor boy was stuffed to the top with feces. No wonder he looked so pale and had a hard time recovering. A little castor oil and all his problems were gone.

Professor Peter Whorwell, a leading expert in gastrointestinal disorders with a specialty IBS unit in the UK, explains in his book Take Control of Your IBS. The complete guide to manage your symptoms that the cause of constipation could also be the cause of a mechanical problem from the puborectalis, a U-shape muscle of the pubic bone that normally keeps the rectum at a certain angle to help to maintain continence. The act of bearing down to pass a bowel movement typically causes this muscle to relax, allowing the rectum to straighten. He doesn't know why, but people with IBS contract their puborectalis and anal sphincter when opening their bowel – "it's like pushing against a closed door". To identify the different types of constipation or diarrhea, you can use the Bristol Stool Chart. Print it out and hang it on the wall of your bathroom, because the information is useful for everyone - especially for children, because they learn to observe their bodies.

Other distressing symptoms of IBS include abdominal bloating and distension. While some people only feel swollen, others actually swell. It is pretty common in IBS-C for a woman to look like she's pregnant when she experiences distension. This condition usually increases during the day, especially after a meal, and subsides overnight. In the past, researchers have considered various possibilities as to why this swelling symptom occurs, among them are psychological stress, excessive or abnormal gas production, motility issues, weakness of abdominal muscles, and abdominal reflex. To shed more light on this issue, Dr. Anurag Agrawal and his research team investigated the relationship between distension and visceral hypersensitivity – an irritation or dysfunction of the intestinal mucosa that can cause you to feel every bit of matter in the rectum. Healthy people do not experience such sensations, but IBS sufferers do. Research shows that people with IBS-D are more likely to experience bloating and visceral hypersensitivity, but not abdominal distension. For people with this set of symptoms it can be worth considering hypnotherapy. Researchers at Monash University in Australia have found that this type of therapy is effective and can even positively influence the central processing of pain responses. Under the chapter 'Mental stress' you will find more information on hypnotherapy.

Distention is common in people with IBS-C, and older people are particularly susceptible. Usually, people with this condition do not suffer from visceral hypersensitivity. Distention can lead to pressure on the bladder and thus to more frequent urination. Some people experience severe pain in the abdomen throughout the day. It seems the stronger the pain, the bigger the belly. Dr. Agrawal research team saw cases where the abdominal circumference was up to 3.9 inch (10 cm) larger than the observed control group. The reason for distention could be an accumulation of feces, leading to the relaxation of the abdominal muscles. It can also be due to excessive intestinal gas produced by bacteria. Professor Whorwell says that distention is more likely to be related to the diaphragm - a muscle that contributes to breathing - that may not contract normally, which also explains why some people experience shortness of breath. He also points out that bloating or distention that does not go up and down throughout the day should be investigated further, as it may not be related to IBS.

In some cases IBS may be caused by a deficiency of serotonin, a hormone responsible for transmitting messages between nerve cells. It is known as the "happy hormone" because it contributes significantly to our sense of wellbeing. It not only affects sleep and mood, but also has a major impact on pain perception and bowel function, especially motility. Serotonin is produced in the gut where bacteria create 95% of the body's requirement and release it into the intestinal walls. A disorder of the serotonin transmitter, a protein that helps to remove this hormone from the gut, can cause this hormone to remain in the intestine, leading to symptoms such as cramps, pain and diarrhea. The link between serotonin and IBS opens up new therapeutic possibilities, as drugs to block or stimulate serotonin receptors may now be able to help.

The low-FODMAP diet is particularly beneficial in relieving symptoms of IBS or acute gastroenteritis. FODMAPs are a group of carbohydrates that are not properly absorbed in the intestines in some people. These carbohydrates can draw water into the small intestine, slow down intestinal motility, and feed bacteria that produce gases as a byproduct. Too much water and gas in the intestine lead to bloated appearance and impaired bowel movements. For some people this diet does not bring the desired result of reducing their symptoms. If this is the case with you, talk to your doctor about prescription medications or try an over-the-counter product such as Iberogast. Be aware that herbal medicines also can cause side effects such as hypersensitivity reactions, skin rash, itching or breathing difficulties. If you suffer from constipation, you can take a laxative, prokinetic agent, dried prunes, or for a short time, a small amount of castor oil to help with bowel emptying. An increased consumption of dietary fiber or a fiber supplement can prevent constipation. For further information on FODMAPs and dietary fiber, see the chapter "Dietary considerations".

Nearly 50% of patients with IBS-D do well on the broad-spectrum, non-absorbable antibiotic rifaximin. It is also prescribed for traveler's diarrhea, liver disease and episodes of hepatic encephalopathy. This medication may not be suitable for pregnant women, as it can harm the fetus. Treating IBS with rifaximin is not a guarantee that symptoms will disappear forever. In the weeks or months following treatment, symptoms may recur. If so, treatment may have to be repeated.

Healing the gut is a complex undertaking and can take much longer than you might imagine. Of course, it is worth looking for short-term solutions that will help you to reduce symptoms and improve your quality of life, but it is even more important to find the root cause of your condition. This may include physical dysfunction, serious illnesses, insomnia, lack of exercise, and chronic stress. In severe cases, it is advisable to work with a multidisciplinary team of health professionals. This can include healthcare providers such as a doctor, physician, gastroenterologist, naturopath, nutritionist, psychologist, or hypnotherapist. If you suffer from IBS-related mental health problems and live in Australia, you can make use of the free mental health service offered by the Royal Melbourne Hospital. If a comprehensive IBS protocol does not result in a life-improving outcome, there is also the option of a fecal microbiome transplant. This intervention is still in its infancy and not a mainstream treatment as it leaves many questions unanswered, such as short- and long-term safety and donor suitability. Initial studies show promising results for gastrointestinal disorders such as IBS.

My experience with doctors is that they struggle with IBS. Their broad medical knowledge and the limited time available for consultation do not allow them to address this condition comprehensively. After I was diagnosed with IBS, I was pretty much on my own. I was offered no treatment, no nutritional explanations, and not even follow-up appointments. It felt like a life sentence that I simply had to accept. Today, I know that I don't have to put up with IBS. After taking care of my health and changing my lifestyle, many of the symptoms I had in the past are no longer present.

# SMALL INTESTINAL BACTERIAL OVERGROWTH

There is much discussion in the media about "good" and "bad" gut bacteria, but this over-simplification does not reflect the fact that a diversity of bacteria and other microbial communities is essential for overall health. Microscopic organisms, such as bacteria, archaea, and yeast, exist everywhere on earth. They have existed for millions of years and have been the only life forms for most of that time. Even today, they are still an integral part of our daily lives and are found in and on our bodies, including the gastrointestinal tract and skin. In the past, science referred to this community of microorganism in the gut as intestinal or gut microflora. This name changed to microbiota as knowledge increased. If one includes the genes of the microorganisms in this ecosystem, it is called the microbiome. Under normal circumstances, microorganisms in the microbiome do not harm us, but there are exceptions. For example, when certain strains grow in the wrong place and in increased numbers. This can lead to a state of imbalance or maladjustment within the microbiome and cause symptoms of indigestion. Such dysbiosis (or dysbacteriosis) can be the cause of many diseases such as SIBO and IBS.

SIBO strongly affects the small intestine. This organ is located between the stomach and the large intestine. Its purpose is the absorption of nutrients and minerals from food. The small intestine is relatively sterile and usually does not house a lot of bacteria, just enough to do its job and protect the body from the wrong kind of microorganism. But if, for whatever reason, the wrong kind of bacteria and other organisms have taken up residence, it will be burdened by them until its function is impaired.

SIBO is neither contagious nor fatal, but it can significantly affect the quality of life. Symptoms can include nausea, flatulence, bloating, abdominal cramps, abdominal pain, constipation and/or diarrhea (the kind of diarrhea that makes you run to the bathroom immediately). Other signs of this condition includes food sensitivities, leaky gut, allergies, inflammation, rosacea, and autoimmune diseases. In severe cases, there is weight loss, nutritional deficiencies (including vitamin B12, vitamin D, and iron), anemia, and steatorrhea. Steatorrhea is the increased excretion of fat in the stool, indicating a fat absorption disorder. The stool floats, smells foul and is lighter than usual. Symptoms of steatorrhea may include a bloated tummy, abdominal pain, or weight loss in adults. When children suffer from this disease, they have difficulty gaining weight. Leaving steatorrhea un-treated may lead to irreversible damage to the pancreas.

Its cause can be physical or structural changes that lead to the stagnation of bacteria in the gastrointestinal tract. Examples are surgery and diverticulitis. The latter disease occurs when pressure is applied to the intestinal lining, causing it to bulge and form small pouches in which bacteria can multiply unhindered, leading to inflammation and swelling. Other causes are decreased acidity in the stomach (hypochlorhydria), so that unwanted microbes or parasites such as *Helicobacter pylori* (*H. pylori*) are not destroyed, or a motility disorder that makes it easy for bacteria to colonize due to inefficient mass transfer. Both decreased acidity and decreased motility are associated with advanced age and female gender.

There are many diseases associated with SIBO, such as celiac disease, multiple sclerosis, diabetes, pancreatic diseases, liver cirrhosis, cystic fibrosis, fibromyalgia. Other conditions may include viral infection, gastroenteritis, food poisoning, multiple use of antibiotics, hormone medications such as birth control pills, alcoholism and the already mentioned IBS. People who suffer from ulcerative colitis, Crohn's disease and disorders of the thyroid, metabolism and immune system are more susceptible to it. There is even an increased risk of developing SIBO due to mold toxicity.

To overcome SIBO, it is highly recommended to consult an experienced healthcare provider who has a special interest in gastrointestinal health. Before you start a treatment, your healthcare provider might recommend that you undergo some medical tests, such as blood and stool tests. With the results, they will be able to draw up a personalized protocol for you. Be patient, as this might take time and money. Don't try to speed up the process by taking supplements because of a "gut feeling" or trend, or a friend who gave you some "good advice". You could make things worse. Each individual body operates so uniquely that something that works for your friend might not work for you; it may even worsen your condition.

## HOW DO YOU KNOW YOU HAVE SIBO?

You cannot conclude that you have SIBO by merely looking at symptoms, such as a bloated tummy, constipation or diarrhea, stomach pain, fatigue, depression, heartburn, or restless legs. The digestive system is so complex that these signs may indicate another condition altogether. For example, IBS has similar symptoms such as constipation or diarrhea, flatulence, abdominal bloating with pain and cramps, or belching. If you experience food sensitivities, headaches, joint pain, fatigue, depression, or issues with your skin, then you might have leaky gut. A deficiency of iron and B12, steatorrhea and weight loss can indicate malabsorption. It is also possible that you have SIBO and other conditions at the same time, or you just have SIBO, or maybe you have neither IBS nor SIBO. To narrow the spectrum of diseases, it is therefore desirable that you have a specific test that indicates or excludes SIBO.

Since SIBO acts in the small intestine, a conventional internal video examination by endoscopy is limited by the nature of the device used. An endoscopy instrument penetrates only a few of centimeters into the first part of the small intestine, while a colonoscopy can only reach a few centimeters into the end part of this organ, so neither procedure can provide a comprehensive picture of the internal situation. Other video techniques involve swallowing a supplement-sized pill with a wireless camera. This procedure is used to investigate gastrointestinal bleeding,

Crohn's disease, polyps and cancer. None of these screening tests are efficient for detecting an overgrowth of bacteria in the small intestine. The most common test to diagnose SIBO is a hydrogen breath test.

## HYDROGEN BREATH TEST

The standard hydrogen breath test for SIBO assesses the production of hydrogen and methane gas in the intestine based on the amount of gas and the transition time. You can purchase a test kit from a lab and perform it at home or at a clinic. There are various hydrogen tests for SIBO on the market but most healthcare providers recommend a 3-hour test. Before you order a test kit, it's worth asking the lab if they will give you a discount for a retest, as you may want to repeat the test at a later stage to check the progress of the treatment. There's usually very little of these gases in the breath. However, when bacteria metabolize carbohydrates, they release gas as a by-product. Some of the gas is absorbed through the intestinal mucosa, excreted as flatulence, or transported into the lungs via the bloodstream. This is where the test comes into play. The breath is collected and analyzed in a laboratory to determine how many bacteria may be present based on their excretion.

The hydrogen breath test for SIBO uses a lactulose and glucose solution to determine this condition. These two solutions can provide information about where bacteria may have settled in the small intestine, as glucose is absorbed mainly in the upper section, and lactulose is absorbed in the last part of this organ. Performing the test can sometimes make symptoms worse. In this case, I recommend you check out Dr. Allison Siebecker's Sibo info website as she offers a fact sheet with suggestions for alleviating these symptoms. She is a luminary in the field of IBS and SIBO.

The result of the SIBO test may show either a methane dominant or hydrogen dominant SIBO. That said, it is not always easy for an inexperienced healthcare provider to interpret test results correctly. Experts in this field are more reliable in their assessment and can also read between the lines of the result to determine if there is a problem with a third gas - hydrogen sulfide. This gas is known to be toxic in high concentrations and affects the gastrointestinal tract. The hydrogen breath test cannot detect this gas.

There are physical differences between people: for some, the small intestine is shorter, for others much longer than commonly thought. These natural variations can affect the test result, as the length of time for the solution to be absorbed is dependent on the length of the intestine. With a 3-hour hydrogen test, you are on the safe side because it covers all varieties of the intestine and also shows a late increase in production of the gases. Scientists believe that the last hour of a 3-hour breath test provides information about the large intestine that also produces hydrogen during digestion.

Diseases that cause carbohydrate malabsorption, such as chronic pancreatitis or celiac disease, may affect the result of the SIBO test. These conditions often lead to a false-negative result because fermentation processes, and thus gas formation, are already out of control. A false-negative result indicates that SIBO is not present, even if it is. Another reason for this result may be slow digestion as it gives a misleading picture of the activity in the intestine. The latter can be counteracted by carrying out the preparatory diet longer than recommended, that is, starting a day or two earlier.

I have done the hydrogen breath test several times. The first time I tested glucose and lactulose to determine the levels of hydrogen and methane gas production in my small intestine. On follow-up tests, and in consultation with my doctor, I just performed the lactulose test to get new data. This procedure has helped me to reduce some of my ongoing costs. However, I would not recommend testing only either lactulose or glucose unless your healthcare provider is very experienced with SIBO, as a misinterpretation of the results can lead to an incorrect treatment.

## HYDROGEN VS METHANE

Hydrogen and methane are produced by microorganisms such as bacteria, fungi, and archaea. Each of these microbes have their favorite food. For example, when you eat certain carbohydrates, refined or natural sugars, you feed specific types of bacteria and fungi. During metabolism, they produce hydrogen, which in turn is a feast for archaea microbes. The tricky part is that these archaea also produce methane as a by-product.

Each of these gases produces different symptoms and requires a different treatment approach, as no two SIBOs are alike. A distinction is made between hydrogen dominant SIBO (D) and methane dominant SIBO (C). The latter condition has recently been renamed as intestinal methanogen overgrowth (IMO) as researchers discovered that an overproduction of methane is not caused by bacteria, but by archaea microbes.

Archaea are the first known living organisms on earth. They formed their very own biochemistry during evolution and are classified as prokaryotes. There are different kinds of archaea: some are heat-lovers who like to live in hot springs; others are salt-lovers and can be found in salt lakes or even in fermented food, like fish sauces. Yet others are found in swamps, sewage treatment facilities and in the guts of cows and humans. These methanogens preferentially feed on hydrogen and carbon dioxide. Since they occur naturally in our gastrointestinal system, they also have a syntrophic relationship with other inhabitants of the microbiome.

## INTESTINAL METHANOGEN OVERGROWTH

In the diverse community of the microbiome, things can sometimes get out of balance. A methanogen with the name *Methanobrevibacter smithii (M. smithii)*, appears to be one of the troublemakers. It was originally thought to be found only in the large intestine, but researchers have proven otherwise and found them recently in the small intestine. In overabundance, this methanogen slows down motility and prolongs transition time. But that's not all, as IMO is also associated with IBS, increased weight, and obesity. When methanogens work in conjunction with hydrogen-producing bacteria, they accelerate the fermentation of carbohydrates, which increases energy production and this can lead to weight gain. A study of animals shows that a high-fat diet triggered the growth of *M. smithii* in all parts of the gastrointestinal tract.

Interestingly, infants cannot produce methane until they are around three years of age. From the age of 14 -18, children have a similar methane production as adults. Even in adulthood not everyone produces hydrogen or methane equally. Some produce only one of these gases. It is also not unusual to see high levels of both gases simultaneously in a SIBO test result.

## HYDROGEN DOMINANT SIBO

Another predominant symptom of SIBO is diarrhea. Bacteria convert food into essential substances such as hydrogen gas, short-chain fatty acids (SCFAs) and carbon dioxide. Normally, this process takes place in the large intestine. But if it happens in the small intestine due to an overgrowth of bacteria in this organ, it can cause irritation and damage to intestinal tissue, leading to leaky gut. There are several theories as to why this may happen. One theory is that increased production of fatty acids is responsible for this intestinal damage. While another theory says that bacteria cause too much water to be drawn into the small intestine, putting pressure on the intestinal walls. Yet another theory is that bile salts are to blame as they can interfere with the absorption of fat and fat-soluble vitamins. Whatever it is, it is not easy to find the exact cause, as it is often a potpourri of conditions.

## HYDROGEN SULFIDE

Besides methane and hydrogen, there is a third troublesome gas called hydrogen sulfide. This gas appears to be linked to diarrhea and urgency as it is a smooth muscle relaxant. Some people experience an alternation with constipation. An indicator of this condition could be that the SIBO test is negative but gastrointestinal problems still exist. Scientific estimates predict that 25% of people suffer from hydrogen sulfide SIBO instead of IMO or SIBO (D).

Since this gas cannot be measured directly with a classic hydrogen breath test, Dr. Pimentel and his team also developed the trio-smart® breath test, produced by Gemelli Biotech. This test can measure all three gases - hydrogen, methane and hydrogen sulfide - which provides a more comprehensive picture of the activity in the gastrointestinal tract. This product can be ordered through your healthcare provider on the Trio-smart website. The preparation and performance of this test is similar to the classic SIBO test, in which a lactulose or glucose solution is ingested.

Let's take a closer look at the world of sulfur and its relatives to better understand what this gas is all about.

## SULFUR, SULFATE, SULFITE

Sulfur is an essential component of life on earth. Whether human, animal, plant, bacteria, or archaea, all living things metabolize sulfur. It is one of the most common minerals in our body and essential for our nerves, bone, and cartilage growth, as well as connective tissue, skin, hair, nails, and the formation of mucus. It supports enzymes, is an antioxidant and is used in the liver detoxification functions. Sulfur content is high in some animal-based foods, such as meat, cheese, cow's milk and hen's eggs, especially the yolk. Plant-based foods such as wine, onions, garlic, broccoli, cauliflower, cabbage, brussels sprouts, kale, and asparagus are all rich sources of this mineral. Sulfur is found in varying quantities in gains and nuts.

When the body metabolizes organic sulfur, it turns into sulfate. According to Dr. Greg Nigh, a naturopathic doctor, oncologist, and the co-founder of Immersion Health, we need constant access to sulfate as it is "gold" for our body. Most sulfates are produced in the intestines or liver, and a shortage of this mineral is associated with a protein deficiency. Proteins are large and complex molecules made up of building blocks called amino acids. There are many, and each of them has its own unique structure and function. Before a protein can fulfil its essential mission in the body, it must form a particular three-dimensional shape. Two sulfur-containing amino acids, methionine and cysteine, play a key role in this process. If sulfate is not formed, proteins cannot fold correctly into the required shapes. This affects the health of the cells and organs. Several things can impair the conversion of sulfur to sulfate. Dr. Nigh mentions that malfunction can be due to a lack of enzyme activity, genetic predisposition, and/or nutrient deficiency. Other causes include the use of chemicals such as Roundup and heavy metals in modern agriculture, as these toxins greatly affect sulfur metabolism. When the body is unable to produce sulfate directly, it tries to get around the problem by making more of two gases: sulfite and hydrogen sulfide.

Hydrogen sulfide has a close relationship with the gastrointestinal system. Many studies focus on its toxic effect, while others on the complementary properties of this molecule. It is a distinct gas with the foul-smell characteristic of rotten eggs. In the right amount, it has a regulating and protecting effect on the gut, but when things get out of balance, this gas can turn against us. Dr. Nirala Jacobi, a naturopathic doctor and an expert in SIBO, explains in one of her podcasts (The SIBO Doctor, episode 34, 2018), that hydrogen sulfide should not be present in the small intestine as it can damage this organ. The large intestine is more robust in this respect, because it can process the gas. She also mentions that people with high levels of hydrogen sulfide gas in their gastrointestinal tract often develop resistance to some antibiotics.

Hydrogen sulfide can affect the heart and act as a neurotoxin, altering the nervous system. Panic attacks and anxiety are just two manifestations of this condition. Other symptoms can include decreased blood pressure, dizziness, brain fog, acne, skin rashes and itching, diarrhea, abdominal pain, urgency, and bloating. It may also have a laxative effect that can lead to dehydration. Menopausal women are more prone to hot flushes due to an overproduction of this gas. One study points out that too much hydrogen sulfide can cause inflammation and damage intestinal tissue, leading to leaky gut syndrome, a condition that is associated with food intolerances and autoimmune diseases. In general, the higher the gas content, the worse the symptoms.

People with ulcerative colitis have a strong tendency to turn sulfur molecules into hydrogen sulfide, which may be responsible for an impaired butyrate metabolism. Butyrate is an essential SCFA that helps to prevent and inhibit bowel cancer, reduce inflammation, improve intestinal motility and visceral hypersensitivity - a hallmark of IBS. Avoiding high-sulfur foods is particularly beneficial for these people, as well as IBS sufferers.

The body is clever at finding ways to compensate if it does not have access to certain essential elements. For example, if your body cannot produce enough sulfate, it produces sulfite instead. This gas also occurs naturally in the body, as it is a by-product of our metabolism. It is not only crucial for the functioning of hormones, but also for connective tissues. Sulfite is present in most common foods and beverages, as well as in acid rain. It is part of the natural fermentation processes, for example in wine and sauerkraut. As a preservative, it is used to inhibit the growth of bacteria and yeasts in a variety of commercial products. Some people are sensitive to sulfite, and may experience severe allergic reactions, such as breathing difficulties, hives, or anaphylactic shock. Dr. Nigh proposes that it can also trigger our sympathetic nervous system, which is responsible for the "fight-or-flight" response. However, if the body is unable to produce the right amount of sulfite it activates the production of hydrogen sulfide instead.

Fortunately, the trio-smart breath test can now measure hydrogen sulfide in the gastrointestinal tract, which was not possible in the past with the conventional hydrogen breath test for SIBO. If you do not have access to the trio-smart test, your healthcare provider can check your SIBO test result. The result might indicate that you suffer from hydrogen sulfide rather than hydrogen or methane gas.

For some SIBO sufferers, avoiding sulfur-containing foods like garlic, eggs, and kale can make a big difference. On the other hand, an exclusively low-sulfur diet means you might not be getting enough of this essential mineral. However, not all unexplained SIBO symptoms are due to hydrogen sulfide. It could also be that you suffer from histamine intolerance, and you may be more prone to headaches and diarrhea. To alleviate these symptoms you can try a variation of Dr. Jacobi's SIBO Bi-Phasic Diet.

## SMALL INTESTINAL FUNGAL OVERGROWTH

Some people with SIBO or IBS also have a small intestinal fungal overgrowth (SIFO); some have all three conditions; others who test negative for SIBO may have SIFO instead. The symptoms of SIFO are similar to those of SIBO and IBS – bloating, indigestion, constipation, diarrhea, and abdominal pain – but also include others such as foggy brain, mood swings, joint pain/discomfort, fatigue, headaches, anxiety and depression. An overwhelming craving for sugar or refined carbohydrates is not unusual. Another sign of this disease is a fungal infection that may be visible on the tongue, vagina, skin, and nails.

People are more susceptible to fungal and yeast infections if they take broad-spectrum antibiotics, regular painkillers, hormone medications such as the contraceptive pill, immunosuppressants, and antacids - including proton pump inhibitors (PPIs). Other risk factors include high levels of stress, excessive alcohol consumption or being over 60 years of age. Certain health conditions are associated with this type of infection, such as autoimmune disease, anemia, diabetes, Ehlers-Danlos syndrome, colectomy, gastrointestinal motility disorder, and low stomach acid.

To gain a better understanding of why SIFO occurs in the body, we have to take a small detour into the realm of fungi. There are around 100,000 different types of organisms within the fungus kingdom, including yeasts, molds, rusts, sooty molds, mildews, and mushrooms. Most of them are quite common in our environment, being found in the ocean, soil, food, and in and on our bodies. Some of these organisms are good for us, like edible mushrooms, while others are not. *Candida* is one of the yeasts that can show up as a white coating on various parts of the body. It can be painful, especially when it occurs in the mouth, where it causes discomfort when swallowing food. Other examples of fungal infections are ringworm, which appears as a circular rash on the skin, and *Aspergillus*, which can be found in people with lung disease.

Another member of the fungal kingdom is mold. There are thousands of different species that reproduce by releasing tiny spores into the air. These tiny particles are not visible to the naked eye. They can be found in moist places such as windows or pipes but also on damp paper and wood. Some mold can even grow in dust, insulation, carpets, on fabrics or food such as grains and nuts. Contact with mold spores can increase the risk of several health issues including chronic respiratory diseases, neurological diseases, and immunological diseases.

Certain molds produce toxins called mycotoxins that can be found in food. One of these toxic chemicals is the highly poisonous aflatoxin. It grows in conditions of high temperature and humidity, such as those found in tropical climates. Many staple foods may be contaminated with this mold during various stages of their production and during storage. This mold is not always visible to the eye as it can penetrate deep into the products. Susceptible foods are wheat, corn, rice, sorghum, tree nuts – pistachio, almond, walnut, coconut, and Brazil nuts – and seeds from which oils are extracted such as soybean, peanut, sunflower, and olives.

Cotton, spices and fruits such as chili peppers, black pepper, coriander, turmeric, ginger, and dried fruits may also be affected. Humans are at risk not only from plant products, but also from animals and their derived products if they have eaten contaminated feed. According to the World Health Organization (WHO), mycotoxins have been linked to long-term health problems such as cancer and failure of the immune system. WHO recommends consuming food that has had minimal storage time, which is mostly the case when fresh fruit and vegetables are purchased locally. If you find any signs of insects, mold, discoloration, damage or shriveling in or on foods, you should not buy or consume it. Eating as diversely as possible reduces the mold intake while promoting a balanced diet. Generally, adults are more tolerant to mycotoxins than children. The good news is that traditionally fermented sauerkraut and tempeh have a protective and eliminating effect on this toxin, as a new study on mice has revealed. The bad news is that fermented foods often aggravate SIBO and IBS symptoms.

SIFO makes you sensitive to products that contain yeasts, such as breads and fermented foods, as the body is already overly stressed with this component. On a low yeast diet, some yeast cells will die because they suffer a nutrient deficiency. Others yeast strains might withstand this adverse condition because they are evolutionarily more adaptable. In this case you might need to take anti-fungal medication such as Nystatin, Fluconazole, Itraconazole or Posaconazole. Be aware that the last three mentioned drugs can interfere with cardiac arrhythmias, blood sugar and anticoagulant medications. Nystatin has few side effects, as only small amounts of it are absorbed into the bloodstream. It acts mainly on the *Candida* fungus, leading to its death. However, Dr. Michael Ruscio, a functional and integrative doctor specializing in gut related disorders, clinical researcher, and author of the book *Healthy Gut, Healthy You. The Personalized Plan to Transform Your Health from the Inside Out*, writes in his online blog that he does not use Nystatin if the fungal overgrowth is in the small intestine. Instead, he likes to use probiotics and herbal antimicrobials such as oregano, artemisia and berberine as they are equally effective in the treatment of fungal infections.

The organic acids test (OAT) is based on the concept that every life form leaves traces of its existence. It can detect abnormally high numbers of fungi, yeasts and bacteria that are present in the body. However, it can't tell where the fungal or bacterial overgrowth is located in the gastrointestinal tract. In addition, this test checks for immune function, causes of fatigue and motility disorders, genetic metabolic abnormalities, vitamins, minerals, oxalates and the presence of toxins. The OAT seems expensive, but it can be worthwhile because your healthcare provider can use the information to design a more tailored treatment plan for you.

Taking a fluid sample from the small intestine via an endoscopy might be a more direct way to check if you have a fungal or yeast problem in this organ. Performing such an invasive procedure for this alone is not recommended, but could be performed if you require endoscopy for other reasons. That's how I did it and my healthcare provider at the time was very happy to get this test result.

> I love chocolate, especially the dark versions, and believed it was good for me as I only consumed it in moderation. Dark chocolate, which may also be gluten and dairy free, not only seems to reduce cardio metabolic disorders, but also provides many minerals, vitamins, and healthy monounsaturated fat. Unfortunately, I had to reevaluate my little pleasure. There are two factors that have led me to stop eating chocolate, even though I find it really hard to resist the temptation. First, it is common for chocolate products to contain mold toxins such as aflatoxin. These mycotoxins can easily develop on cocoa beans – if, for example, the beans were damaged by insects or have not been handled properly during harvesting and storage. It is tricky to know which chocolate contains mycotoxin and which does not, so I prefer to stay away from it. The other issue with chocolate is that it can cause constipation, especially in people with IBS-C. The reason for this may lie in the high fat, sugar, and caffeine content. I can confirm this, because all I have to do is take one look at chocolate and I have problems with bowel movements.

# SIBO TREATMENT

Overcoming SIBO depends on whether your condition is already chronic, if the underlying conditions have been identified, and if the treatment is working. Although current treatments for SIBO have been refined in recent years, there is still a long way to go before a simplified method that will help most cases is found.

Please, do not self-medicate. The use of dietary supplements, essential oils, and herbal blends requires a thorough knowledge of their use, quantity, and origin. Many people overdose while thinking they are doing something good for themselves. In fact, you could harm yourself, causing internal pain and damage to your intestine. Ultimately, you will never know what kind of chemical compound you are creating in your body when you mix all kinds of supplements and herbs together. Instead, consult a naturopath who is knowledgeable about gastrointestinal diseases as they are trained to find the right tinctures, doses and times to take them for your condition. Don't be tempted to go to the herbalist around the corner for a solution to SIBO and IBS. You will waste your time and money, as they will not have a comprehensive clinical picture of your health.

> I once made the terrible mistake of following an advice I found on the internet. I tried oregano oil because I thought it would help me with SIBO. After taking the recommended dose listed on the bottle, I had terrible, burning pain in my stomach for many hours and almost collapsed. So, please don't do it. If you want to try something you've heard might help, do it under the supervision of your healthcare provider.

A SIBO treatment is usually divided into different stages – each has a specific focus. The first aims to provide rapid relief of symptoms. The next attempts to combat the overgrowth in the small intestine. In parallel, the cause of this condition is sought. Finally, the focus is on stabilizing health outcomes.

## STAGE ONE

At the beginning of the treatment, laboratory tests are usually carried out to get an overview of your general health. Depending on who you consult, for example a doctor or naturopath, different tests may be performed. The doctor would ask for some standard tests to determine that there are no serious diseases behind your symptoms. They may order stool and blood tests that are covered by the public healthcare system. If your doctor finds nothing significant wrong with you, they may advise you to take a laxative or refer you to a specialist. Often, the search for an answer to your problems ends here because the healthcare system is not designed to find the root causes of elusive conditions like SIBO and IBS.

When you start your journey with a naturopath, they also order tests. However, their functional tests differ from those from the doctor. They are usually not covered by the healthcare system or private health insurance and are quite costly. It can be useful to have these tests done as they provide information about metabolic processes, genetics, hormone balance, the gastrointestinal tract, and dietary needs. To save money, you can have the standard blood and stool tests done by your doctor and pass the results on to your naturopath. Adding only a few functional tests may be enough to provide a comprehensive picture of your health. If antibiotics are required, you may need to get the script from your doctor as in some countries a naturopath can prescribe only natural medicines such as vitamins, minerals, and herbal remedies.

To combine the benefits of the two medical worlds mentioned above, you can see a doctor who specializes in functional medicine or integrative medicine. They have completed medical training but have additional expertise, for example, in naturopathy. This knowledge helps them more easily identify and understand causes of the disease. These doctors can order standard and functional tests and know how to interpret them. They may also charge higher consultation fees that are not necessarily covered by the healthcare system. You should be aware that cost can become quite overwhelming when you add up consultation fees, functional tests, treatments and supplements.

In this first stage, a diet such as the low-FODMAP diet or the SIBO Bi-Phasic Diet by Dr. Jacobi is usually introduced to alleviate symptoms. The idea behind these diets is to reduce the fermentation of carbohydrate in the small intestine while increasing the absorption of nutrients. People with SIBO are often deficient in vitamins, especially fat-soluble vitamins, minerals, and proteins. They also tend to suffer from carbohydrate malabsorption. Part of the SIBO treatment can include nutritional and digestive support to restore the intestinal lining.

## STAGE TWO

The next stage focuses on treating the overgrowth in the small intestine and stabilizing the motility of the gastrointestinal tract. The eradication of bacteria is usually achieved by an antimicrobial agent, which can be either a pharmaceutical or herbal product. There are two theories underlying this process. The first says that it is best to maintain the usual diet during treatment. Feeding bacteria with carbohydrates prevents them from going into hibernation and thus escaping the treatment agent. This approach may work well for a short one or two-week course of antibiotics but may not work for an herbal antimicrobial option since this may take several weeks or months. The second theory is that one should start a special diet a few weeks before the treatment to eliminate bacteria. This approach allows the microbiome to slowly adjust to fewer carbohydrates and prevents gut bacteria from going into hibernation. It should also reduce the side effects that occur when microbes die, called "die-off". Endotoxins are released during the elimination of bacteria, parasites, and yeast. These are specific carbohydrates (glycoconjugates) that trigger pro-inflammatory reactions and activate the immune system. During this process you may experience flu-like symptoms such as fever, muscle aches, runny nose, fatigue, and headaches. In medical terms these "die-off" symptoms are called Jarisch-Herxheimer reactions. Not only antimicrobial, anti-fungal or anti-parasitic treatments can trigger them, but also an elimination diet, elemental diet, or an increased intake of probiotics. To alleviate these symptoms, your healthcare provider may recommend supportive supplements or anti-inflammatory foods. Drink plenty of warm water throughout the day and get enough rest.

To determine whether the antimicrobial treatment is successful, a retest for SIBO is usually performed. If the result is satisfactory, a prokinetic agent is added to the treatment plan. This agent supports the migrating motor complex (MMC) to prevent constipation and SIBO relapses. It is recommended to take this agent for up to six months to ensure proper bowel function. During this phase, foods are reintroduced into the diet. This must be done slowly and selectively to avoid inflammation and worsening of symptoms. If you also have SIFO, an antifungal herb or medication will be given.

I have successfully taken Iberogast and MotilPro for many months. However, I was tired of taking large amounts of supplements every day, so I looked for alternative options. Since the active ingredient in MotilPro is ginger extract, I switched to fresh ginger. Ginger is an amazing root plant that is one of the most health-promoting spices in the world. Among its many benefits, it supports metabolism, muscle function, and the heart. It helps with headaches, nausea, motion sickness, and high LDL cholesterol. As if that were not enough, it also reduces inflammation, gas and bloating, while strengthening the digestive system. With all these benefits, it is not surprising that it has found its way into so many medicines and cuisines around the world.

## ANTIMICROBIALS

Antimicrobials are an important component when it comes to eradicating bacteria. These may be pharmaceutical or herbal products. For example, rifaximin is often prescribed for SIBO (D), IBS, dysbiosis, travelers' diarrhea, and liver diseases. It is a nonabsorbable antibiotic that does not enter the bloodstream and therefore considered safe. It seems that it does not create a favorable environment for yeast growth.

Rifaximin alone may not be as effective if you suffer from IMO. In this case, it is combined with another antibiotic such as neomycin. Although these antibiotics form a good partnership, neomycin should be used with caution because it has a long list of side effects. Other systemic antibiotics you may be offered include tetracyclines and metronidazole. I would recommend becoming familiar with antibiotics and discuss any concerns with your doctor. There are alternative treatments if you are not comfortable with them. Taking an antibiotic is no guarantee of overcoming SIBO forever. Studies show that recurrences of the disease within a year is quite common.

An herbal antimicrobial treatment can be as effective as antibiotic treatment. I would recommend you consult a naturopath with expertise in SIBO and IBS as they can find the right herbs for you. Even though naturopathic herbs sound natural and safe, they can be potent and powerful. They are actually drugs that use an active ingredient from a plant. Don't confuse them with dietary supplements, as these usually provide minerals and vitamins to compensate for nutrient deficiencies. In daily use, herbs are used only in small quantities to season meals or create fragrances. You would not add cloves in high quantities to your food, would you?

Be wary if someone advises you to use an antimicrobial herbal treatment for an extended period; Dr. Ruscio points out that overuse may lead to a *Clostridium difficile* infection. Symptoms can range from diarrhea to a life-threating inflammation in the colon. Usually, this bacterium is found in elderly people in hospitals or care facilities, but it may also occur after taking antibiotic medication.

Antibiotics or herbal medicines do not address the root cause of SIBO, IBS or other digestive disorders. At worst, they upset the microbiome by eliminating not only unwanted but also beneficial microbes, and this can be the cause of diseases such as obesity and insulin resistance. There is no right or wrong in the process of healing from SIBO – for some people, antibiotics seem to do the job; for others, herbal options are more effective. It is all about preferences, responses, and success rate, as well as cost and availability.

## STAGE THREE

This last stage is not always clearly separable from the previous one, as each protocol is tailored to the individual needs of the patient. Nevertheless, the goal here is to find the underlying causes of SIBO if they have not already been considered. This may be parasites, toxins, physical dysfunction, food poisoning, or celiac disease. It is medical detective work that can take a lot of time and may be quite costly. The individual's lifestyle is considered because it can provide clues as to the underlying causes. Poor diet, alcohol consumption, lack of or excessive exercise, sleep issues, stress and mental health are the focus here.

During this stage, the diet is expanded, and probiotics are included to promote the growth of beneficial microorganisms in the gastrointestinal tract. There are different views on the use of probiotics in SIBO and IBS treatment. One notion is that adding bacteria to the already existing overgrowth in the small intestine can be counterproductive and worsen symptoms. Another view is that the introduction of these helpers is an essential part of the self-healing process. Yet another opinion is that it just depends on the right timing and the right probiotic to be integrated into the treatment.

Once established in the microbiome, probiotic organisms produce SCFAs and help regulate neurological functions and the endocrine system, which includes the thyroid and adrenal glands. Probiotics also play an important role in healing the gut mucosa and restoring gut motility. On the negative side, probiotics may trigger symptoms such as bloating, fullness and brain fog in some people because they have the potential to produce additional methane gas and therefore carry an increased risk of worsening symptoms.

Be cautious when purchasing over-the-counter probiotics. Check the ingredients on the label as dietary supplements are not considered drugs and are therefore not regulated by the Food and Drug Administration. This means there is uncertainty about the quality, purity, and viability of the bacterial strains in these products. Many of these supplemental products use fillers like tapioca or potato starch, lactose, pectin, inulin, carrageenan, or other ingredients that can make symptoms worse. Also, the capsules of these supplements may be made of gelatin from beef or pork of unspecified origin. If you are like me, you may react to one of these substances and new symptoms may appear. Keep in mind if you have a "the more the better" attitude when it comes to supplementation, the results will not necessarily be superior. It is important to know what the body really needs and in what quantity to support its self-healing powers.

I have made a habit of looking at the ingredient list of all my supplements and medications because I have had nasty surprises in the past. Once my doctor recommended that I should go on a dairy-free diet but at the same time suggested a supplement that contained lactose. Another time, I received a compounded product from my pharmacy that contained a lactose filler. Upon request, they changed the formula and squeeze the ingredients into small capsules without fillers. Since puberty, I can't tolerate pork products – they give me lots of pimples. During my SIBO treatment, I had a terrible skin and didn't know why. After discarding all the capsules of the supplements and taking only their contents, my skin cleared up immediately. I concluded that some of the capsules must have been made from pork gelatin.

Since the microbial colonization in the gut is rather individual because it is influenced by diet, lifestyle, and environment, it is not easy to guess what type of probiotic or foods will be helpful for each of us. The fact that there are hundreds of probiotic supplements on the market does not make it easy to make the right choice. Dr. Ruscio recommends looking for a multispecies probiotic, as these are well researched for IBS. He recommends choosing products that have a high number of colony-forming units, ideally in the billions, and probiotic species clearly labeled. He also says that it is best to choose a brand that has good manufacturing practices and displays a manufacturing and/or expiry date. Certification of the probiotic species by independent laboratory analysis is another positive indicator for the product.

There is a lot of talk in today's media about probiotics and prebiotics, but it is not always clear to everyone what the difference between them is. Therefore, let's dive a little deeper into this subject to help you make informed choices.

## PREBIOTICS, PROBIOTICS AND POSTBIOTICS

Although these terms sound similar, each plays a unique role. Simply said, probiotics are living microorganism that are beneficial to the host, while prebiotics are the food source for the gut microbiome. Postbiotics are the wholesome final products, also known as SCFAs, that result when the gut micro-organisms have nibbled on the prebiotics.

The diverse community of microorganisms in the large intestine cannot survive or thrive if they are not properly nourished. They need food like onions, garlic, bananas, chicory root and Jerusalem artichoke. Prebiotic foods resist digestion in the small intestine, so that micro-organisms in the large intestine can benefit from them. Most of these foods share common features: they contain non-digestible fiber and plant-derived carbohydrates called oligosaccharides - oligos for short. Oligos are a variety of simple sugar molecules that favor the growth of bacteria that are important for maintaining gut health.

Unlike prebiotics, probiotics are the living microorganisms that are used to supplement the microbiota and help to regulate the immune system. Although probiotic strains such as *Lactobacillus* and *Bifidobacterium* are known to play an important part in the treatment of many diseases, how they work is still a mystery. Scientists have discovered that they are especially supportive of the large intestine, but to reach this area they have to overcome some life-threatening obstacles. For example, after swallowing probiotic capsules, the strains they contain must first survive the harsh acidic environment of the stomach and be resistant to gastric juices and digestive enzymes. Then, further down the digestive tract, they are confronted with other microbes that do not like new intruders. However, if they are lucky and manage to reach the desired location, they can start to colonize the microbiome. Once established, they help to reduce inflammation as well as symptoms associated with autoimmune diseases, allergies, asthma, inflammatory bowel disease, celiac disease, rheumatoid arthritis, multiple sclerosis, thyroid disease, leaky gut, depression, and chronic fatigue.

The *Bifidobacterium* family is one of the first strains to enter the body after birth. These guys help us tolerate a sugar molecule called lactose, which is found in breast milk and dairy products. Studies have shown that breastfed babies have a good percentage of *Bifidobacteria* in their gut, which arms them against infection. People with lactose intolerance and food allergies may benefit from taking *Bifidobacterium longum* to improve tolerance to small amounts of dairy products. Its sibling, *Bifidobacterium lactis*, boosts immunity and assists with digestive diseases. It can also help to fight salmonella bacteria and relieve associated diarrhea.

Nowadays, there is a whole range of probiotic supplements on the market. Especially those that promote SCFA production, such as the *Bifidobacterium* and *Lactobacillus* strains. These supplements have their place after antibiotic therapy to restore the microbial community in the gut. The question is whether these supplements are beneficial for all of us. A study notes that taking probiotics is associated with an increase of methanogen bacteria and may not be a favorable treatment for predominately constipation symptoms as seen in IMO. Some of the probiotic strains have been associated with an increased mortality in patients with severe acute pancreatitis. Moreover, widely accepted probiotics such as *Lactobacillus spp.* may cause infections in people who are immunocompromised and/or have intestinal diseases. Although the likelihood that probiotics pose a health risk is very low, it cannot be ignored.

Before capsules and supplements ruled our lives, there were many common probiotic foods on our plates. Each traditional cuisine has its own favorites, whether it is sauerkraut, kombucha, kefir, apple cider vinegar, miso, tempeh, kimchi, pickles, sourdough bread, or even certain cheeses. These dishes often arose from the need to preserve a harvest. By using fermentation techniques and naturally occurring bacteria, yeasts, molds, and fungus from the environment, humans discovered how to convert sugars and starches into lactic acid - the lacto-fermentation was born. This process not only preserves food but also promotes beneficial bacteria, enzymes, B vitamins, and omega-3 fatty acids. When incorporating fermented foods into your diet, try to use raw and unpasteurized products to get the full probiotic benefit from them. Don't be tempted to buy commercial products as they are usually pasteurized or heat-treated. This kind of procedure kills the beneficial bacteria and enzymes that we actually want to ingest. Keep your fermented products in the fridge and take them out in time so that they can develop their full flavor before adding them to a meal. Be a little cautious if you integrate them into your diet. Observe your body and check if symptoms intensify. It may be necessary to reduce the overgrowth in the small intestine first before you can enjoy the benefits of fermented foods.

Yogurt is a well-known probiotic and the result of a fermentation process. There is a big difference between traditional fermentation techniques and today's industrially manufactured products. Some commercial yogurts claim to have health benefits, but studies show that this is not always the case. They do not always achieve the desired result of positively influencing the microbiome. Some of these products even have a negative impact on carbohydrate metabolism, and yet others contain no bacteria strains at all. At their best, cultured dairy products contain a bacterium called *Lactobacillus acidophilus* that can help to maintain cholesterol levels and balance the microbiome. Women in particular can benefit from this bacterium because it helps fight off vaginal yeast infections. Other strains like *Lactobacillus plantarum* and *Lactobacillus brevis* help to accelerate protein digestion, which is important for the prevention of food intolerances.

On the internet there are numerous recipes for making homemade yogurt from dairy, or alternative ingredients such as coconut milk. What they all have in common is that they require a yogurt starter culture. If you want to use dairy, try to use milk that still contains healthy natural bacteria as in organic, or biodynamic milk. If you have issues with the lactose in milk, ferment your homemade yogurt for twenty-four hours or longer (depending on your taste) as this process makes it virtually lactose-free. If you have a very sensitive gut or are starting a Specific Carbohydrate Diet, you might like to buy a culture that does not contain *Bifidobacterium* strains because it can easily take over in the intestine and may cause health problems. These cultures might be a bit more expensive, but you need only a tiny amount to make a homemade yogurt; any remaining culture can be frozen and thawed in portions as needed. Depending on how often you make yogurt, it can take months to use it up, so it's worth the money.

Ayurveda is a traditional Indian system of medicine, well-known for its health approaches to digestive problems. From an Ayurvedic perspective, it is not recommended to eat or drink cold yoghurt, or to combine it with fresh fruit, as both make digestion more difficult. It is best to use plain yogurt diluted with some warm water as a digestive aid at the end of or between meals. For this purpose, mix about a quarter of a cup of yogurt (preferably homemade) with a few pinches of ginger and cumin powder in a glass. Pour warm (not hot!) water over it. Stir it until it forms a watery milky drink, known as "lassi". Alternatively, use a blender or immersion hand blender to achieve a smooth consistency.

To maintain the beneficial effects of probiotics, these little guys must be continuously added to your microbiome. As soon as you stop, the microbiome can return to its previous state within a couple of weeks. To avoid adding unnecessary or wrong bacterial strains, it is desirable to know which bacteria and yeasts your body is missing. A naturopath can initiate a comprehensive stool test that evaluates the gastrointestinal microbiome by focusing on inhabitants, digestion and absorption, inflammation, as well as metabolic indicators. These tests are quite expensive but can provide further information on your overall health, and whether you may need to pay special attention to certain nutritional factors. I did the GI Effects® stool profile test from Genova Diagnostics, which I was able to order through my naturopath. Alternatively, you could volunteer to be a subject in a research study of the American Gut Project and British Gut Project and donate your stool to the scientific community. These projects are part of the much larger Earth Microbiome Project that involves over a hundred labs worldwide. The test is cheaper, currently by donation, which is reflected in a less detailed result and a longer waiting time for the result. However, due to the Covid pandemic, these laboratories may be overloaded with more urgent activities and may not offer their service at the moment.

A note of caution: Fermented foods, aged cheese, vinegar, bone broth, cured meats and refrigerated leftovers contain higher levels of histamines, a chemical found in our cells that sometimes causes symptoms of allergies such as a runny nose or sneezing. Histamine intolerance is often associated with a dysfunctional gut and SIBO. You'll find more information on histamines in the chapter "Histamine, oxalates and salicylates".

> As a German I love sauerkraut, but it made my symptoms worse. My friend Anna, who owned a sauerkraut business, advised me to start slowly, adding only a small amount to main meals and mixing it thoroughly with the other ingredients on my plate. As an alternative, she suggested I could drink a

teaspoon of the fermented juice instead. Encouraged by her advice, I regularly consumed a small amount of sauerkraut juice a few weeks after my antimicrobial treatment. Today I can tolerate small portions of fermented foods without problems.

## BIOFILM

After a successful treatment of SIBO or IBS, symptoms usually return in a few weeks or months. One of the reasons for this phenomenon is biofilms in your gut. Biofilms are everywhere. They are found in every environment on living and non-living surfaces. They are in the kitchen drain as well as in our body. You may have heard of plaque – the sticky, colorless film on teeth that can cause cavities and gum disease – this is also a biofilm. A biofilm provides shelter for microorganisms and is made of a gel-like matrix of DNA, proteins, and polysaccharides. Microorganisms can form a diverse community with a complex communication system within a biofilm. They can adapt to lower nutrient requirements, hide from the immune system and can even influence it. Not all biofilms are harmful, but the more destructive ones can promote inflammation and nutritional deficiency. The host may suffer from psychological and physical problems as seen in inflammatory bowel diseases, prostate infections, and Barrett's esophagus. The list of recognized diseases caused by biofilms and their inhabitants is not limited to the gut; in fact, researchers have found that people with periodontal problems are more likely to develop heart disease and strokes because the biofilm in their mouth spreads into their circulatory system.

Obtaining a biofilm sample in the gastrointestinal tract is a difficult task because the biofilm intermingles with the intestinal matrix. Sometimes it can be detected during an endoscopy - but it may also be induced by this procedure, for example, from clinical detergents, manual cleaning, and incomplete drying of instruments. Even if the clinician could obtain a sample of a biofilm from a swab, stool or urine test, it is very hard to distinguish between the pathogens and the healthy microbial community in a culture environment.

Targeting the microorganisms under the biofilm with antibiotics is a difficult task because they are shielded from this treatment. Besides the microorganisms that colonize, there are also individual, independent planktonic bacteria that like to swim around in the body fluid causing trouble, which makes things even more complicated. Researchers point out that it is almost impossible to eliminate the inhabitants of the biofilm, even if they are treated with a high dose of antibiotics. These microorganisms are only temporarily weakened and are then able to re-form and repair the thin layer of biofilm to protect themselves again. Within a few months, they will return to their original state, only this time possibly in a more antibiotic-resistant form. To counteract this effect, it is advisable to add beneficial bacteria and yeasts to the micro-biome by incorporating pre- and probiotics into your diet.

My doctor thought that my SIBO relapses were caused by biofilm and recommended seeing a practitioner trained in a visceral manipulation method (barralinstitute.com.au). This technique gently massages and manipulates individual organs. Not only did it help me with my bladder problem, but I think it did a good job of clearing some biofilm in my intestines. The practitioner was able to feel the biofilm adhering to the intestinal mucosa and detached it using a special technique. He warned me that I might experience die-off symptoms after this treatment. He was right – the next day I felt as if I had the flu. If you want to try this technique, it is recommended to undergo an antimicrobial treatment at the same time, so that the released bacteria are simultaneously eliminated.

# CONCEPT SUMMARY

» Microorganisms such as bacteria, fungi and archaea are natural components of our environment and thus of our gastrointestinal tract. An imbalance of these organisms in the gut can lead to an overgrowth or reduction of certain species, resulting in diseases such as SIBO and IBS.

» SIBO and IBS are neither contagious nor fatal, but they can severely impair the quality of life. If untreated, they may lead to health issues such as leaky gut, food sensitivities, allergies, inflammation, and autoimmune diseases.

» SIBO and IBS are associated with many disorders, whether as cause, effect, or in co-existence. At first sight it is difficult to distinguish these conditions from each other, or even from more severe diseases such as inflammatory bowel disease, because symptoms are very similar. It is common for SIBO and IBS to occur simultaneously. It seems that these two conditions stimulate each other.

» IBS is not easy to pin down, as testing options for this condition are limited. Usually, the complexity of the symptoms and the exclusion of other diseases lead to the diagnosis of IBS. The ibs-smart test offers another way to diagnose this condition.

» A SIBO treatment is usually carried out in various stages and may include antimicrobials, prokinetic agents, nutritional supplements, probiotics, dietary and lifestyle changes. However, recurrence of SIBO after treatment is common.

» An overgrowth of fungi in the small intestine is often accompanied by diseases such as SIBO and IBS. It must be treated at the same time. Treatment of fungal infection leads to improvement of gastrointestinal symptoms.

» Biofilm, a protective shield under which microorganisms such as bacteria and fungi hide, can hinder the healing process in the intestinal healing journey and may be the cause of disease recurrence.

# THE DIGESTIVE SYSTEM

Our body is in constant communication with us, but most of the time we do not understand its language. It's so easy to take its functionality for granted, especially when everything seems to be running smoothly. But there are moments when we suppress or ignore its subtle signals until things go awry. That's why it's so important to build a close relationship with our bodies. A first step is to get to know its functions. That way, you can better understand your symptoms and make the right choices to alleviate them.

A dysfunctional digestive system not only affects the rest of the body but also impacts our daily lives. The digestive system is a group of organs that convert food into usable components to sustain the functions of the body. For this reason, it works tirelessly day and night to support, maintain and repair the body. Some of its everyday jobs include regulating the immune system, building hormones, and governing a population of 100 trillion microorganism. Even when we are asleep, it is busy doing something. Today's scientists believe that the gastrointestinal system is our second brain because it has its own complex nervous system - the enteric nervous system - which communicates extensively with the brain; hence the term "gut-brain axis".

The gut analyzes everything we put in our mouths or on our skin. This information is then passed on to the brain to make decisions on how to work with these substances. Every happy relationship is based on good communication, and in the case of the gut-brain axis, the vagus nerve serves as a messenger. It is the second largest nerve in the entire body and touches most organs, such as the heart, lungs, digestive tract, and genitals. If this nerve is stressed for prolonged periods, for example by poor posture, alcohol, or spicy food, it can become inflamed. It can also be severely damaged by radiation therapy or head injury. A strained vagus nerve can cause gastrointestinal problems, fatigue, anxiety, and depression. As in any relationship, miscommunication can lead to malfunction and tension. This is just as true for the gut-brain relationship. Care of the vagus nerve facilitates good communication.

## MOUTH, EYES AND NOSE

But let's start where digestion is first stimulated. The sight and smell of food triggers this process. Whether you are doing the grocery shopping, preparing food, or having the meal in front of you, digestion starts its course. These first impressions of food are transmitted to the brain. If the food is perceived as safe and appetizing, the brain sends impulses to different parts of the digestive system. These signals stimulate the saliva production, contract the stomach, and induce the digestive glands to produce and store secretions. These secretions are then directed into the digestive tract to assist digestion and absorption of food. You can support this process by taking time to explore the food you want to eat. Make sure the food will not cause any problems and make you sick. Is it tasty, does it smell and look good? Use not only your eyes, but also your sense of smell in this exploration.

The interplay between the teeth, mastication muscles, tongue, and taste buds is remarkable. After the brain has approved the food, the teeth start chewing, the tongue plays around, and the mouth closes. The food is mushed and mixed with the saliva. This versatile, watery substance has antibacterial compounds and various enzymes to break down and moisten the food for a better swallow. Saliva is an essential component of a healthy digestive system, as it protects the cells of the stomach and the mucosa of the esophagus. The salivary glands are responsible for the production of this precious salivary fluid. You can support this process by chewing your food well and eating in a quiet and relaxing environment, which will also help to reduce bloating. Interestingly, event-related stress, as it is experienced in sports activities, can increase the concentration of salivary proteins. This is also true when the body is calm and relaxed, because here too the salvia is richer in protein and the blood vessels around the glands are strengthened. On the other hand, inflammation, and infection, as well as chronic psychological stress, can lead to negative changes in the components of this fluid and its flow.

Most compounds of the blood are found in the saliva too, but in a different concentration. A non-invasive and inexpensive saliva test can give valuable indications of general health and disease. This test can also show a more complete picture of unbound, bioavailable hormones in the body. For people who can't undertake a blood test, a saliva test might be a good alternative.

The sensory receptors of the tongue can detect five basic tastes. These are sweet, salty, sour, bitter and umami, which is a savory taste. Each flavor signals a different approach to the food at hand. Is it safe, or dangerous? We first experienced the sweet taste through our mother's milk, which conditioned us from an early age to classify it as pleasing and safe. In contrast, bitter and sour flavors are often associated with harmful chemicals. Studies have shown that the role of receptors in the mouth goes beyond taste alone. People who can easily identify different bitter substances have a stronger immune system than people who can't.

Bitter substances stimulate and promote digestive enzymes. They not only nourish wanted bacteria but also help to ward off unwanted strains. They can even prevent microorganisms from forming protective biofilms. Unlike traditional cultures that use bitters to aid the digestive system, it seems that the modern Western diet neglects this flavor in favor of the much more popular sweet and salty tastes. China, India, and Southeast Asia integrate bitters in their cuisine every day. While in Europe and South America people like to drink bitter drinks after a heavy meal. Also, in the traditional Ayurveda medicine, it is recommended to take some bitter herbs before meals to stimulate digestion. When you incorporate vegetables such as chicory, dandelion, and bitter melon into your diet, you're not only doing something for your health but you're also tapping into a new world of pleasurable tastes. It is best to gradually introduce bitters into meals, as the taste buds need time to get used to them. Use caution when using bitters if you have problems with heartburn, as they can increase the acidity in the stomach and make symptoms worse.

Oral health is more than just brushing your teeth twice or three times a day; it can prevent many diseases and reduce premature mortality. Regular dental check-ups may help to identify signs of nutritional deficiencies, infections, immune disorders, injuries, or oral cancer. The WHO points out in its 2003 oral health report that oral infections can kill. Even mild infections can threaten overall health as they affect the entire body. People with a weakened immune system are more at risk. Therapies and medications are common triggers for compromised functionality and health of the mouth. Be vigilant – if you notice any changes in your oral health, don't hesitate to talk to your dentist or healthcare provider about it.

## GASTROINTESTINAL CANAL

The gastrointestinal system is a continuous hollow muscular tube with four tissue layers. The mucosa is the inner surface layer that serves as a barrier between the outside and inside world. Its mucosal properties prevent viruses, bacteria, or fungi from entering the body. At the same time, it stops the body tissues from becoming dehydrated. Within the mucosa there is a thin layer, the muscularis mucosae, that is responsible for local movement. Scientists now know that this thin layer is essential for a healthy gut. Dysfunction of its motor activity leads to chronic inflammatory bowel disease. Directly under the mucosa is a supporting layer, the submucosa, which is connected to the blood vessels of the mucosa. Macronutrients, vitamins, and minerals circulate through the body via these blood vessels. The submucosa provides strength and helps the gastrointestinal organ resist excessive stretching, distension, and tearing. The last two layers, the muscularis and the serosa, perform a kind of rhythmic wave contraction, peristalsis, which moves food along and lubricates the intestine, so that it does not rub against the surrounding muscles and bones. All these layers contain large amounts of collagen.

Collagen is the most common protein in mammals and makes up a third of the human body mass. It gives elasticity to the skin, supports the joints. It is also an important resource for the wound-healing process because it helps to keep wounds sterile and fight infections. As we age, the production of collagen slows down and the elasticity of cells is no longer maintained. A consequence of this process is the degradation of the skin and the formation of wrinkles.

Our body can produce collagen naturally from protein sources such as meat, eggs, cheese, legumes, beans, algae, or quinoa. There are about twenty-nine members of the collagen family, which are divided into several groups according to their structure. It is worth noting that collagen contains a high proportion of the amino acid hydroxyproline, which is not found in other proteins. On the other hand, it does not contain tryptophan, one of the nine essential amino acids. Other amino acids in collagen are glycine and proline, both of which play an important role in digestive health. These two amino acids not only support the gastrointestinal tract, but are also vital for the nervous and immune systems.

Vitamin C supports the synthesis of collagen, as do zinc and sulfur. Together, they act as antioxidants by preventing oxidative stress. Vitamin C is found in citrus fruits, peppers, and tomatoes, while sulfur is found in broccoli, onions, and garlic. Foods containing zinc include red meat, poultry, some types of seafood, dairy products, beans, whole grains, and nuts. A balanced diet with a variety of plant foods throughout the day ensures an adequate supply of amino acids, as well as vitamins and minerals.

The food industry uses gelatin, which contains collagen, as a texturizer to stabilize products and enhance the taste experience because it helps to gently release flavors. It is widely used in products such as yogurt, ice cream, jelly (Jell-O), and gummy bears. It is also found in capsules used for medications and dietary supplements. Pure gelatin is a tasteless animal product made from bones, skin, and cartilage. It dissolves slowly in the body and can be easily absorbed because its amino acids have already been broken down. But stop, before running into the nearest supermarket or health food store to buy some gelatin products or collagen powder to support your gut health. Think again. Many such products can worsen symptoms or cause even more damage in the gut because they may contain high levels of sugar and additives. Avoid these and look for products that come from grass-fed animals and organic farming. This way, you are avoiding toxins, hormones, antibiotics, and pesticides that come with factory farming. Quality starts with agriculture and animal welfare.

For natural soothing and restoration of the mucosa and to help with constipation, my Ayurvedic practitioner recommended a special tea to me. It is made from mucilaginous herbs like marshmallow and licorice roots and a small amount of slippery elm bark powder. When I started drinking this prebiotic tea I immediately felt a relief in my gut. The result was a picture-book stool. It also helped with my skin and reduced irritation caused by certain foods. These herbs should not be taken in the first phase of the SIBO treatment, as this prebiotic can increase the growth of bacteria. There is no special rule – you can try it and see whether it helps or hinders your healing process. To brew this tea, you need some shredded marshmallow and licorice roots. Take 2 tablespoons of each and soak them overnight in around 54 ounces (1.6 liters or 6 cups) of water. In the morning, boil down the liquid to about 16 ounces (500 ml). Strain the tea through a sieve and discard the roots. Add half a teaspoon of slippery elm bark powder to a cup of the tea and drink it fifteen minutes before the main meals. The tea keeps in the fridge for up to four days. Dr. John Douillard, an ambassador for traditional Ayurvedic medicine and advocate for eating seasonal local products, offers a slightly different recipe and method on his Lifespa website. His method is to drink a tablespoon of the tea throughout the day, or at least every two hours and before and after meals. He recommends keeping a day's supply in a jar near you and storing the rest in the refrigerator.

## ESOPHAGUS AND STOMACH

The esophagus connects the pharynx and the stomach. It has an upper and lower valve to allow partially digested, chewed food to pass from the mouth to the stomach and prevent it from moving back up. If you suffer from reflux, it is likely that the lower valve is not working well. Small amounts of food with some stomach acid pushes back into the esophagus. The result is heartburn. If this reflux occurs regularly, the stomach acid will eventually damage the lining of this tube. This condition can lead to diseases such as Barrett's esophagus and gastroesophageal reflux disease (GERD). Both must be addressed professionally.

The stomach holds and processes food for a few hours. Without this storage, we would have to eat constantly to keep the body happy. Its powerful mechanical and chemical tools for digestion are a combination of muscle contractions and an acidic mixture of gastric juices which make the stomach environment acidic. One of the functions of the gastric juices is to convert chemicals like pepsinogen into the digestive enzymes pepsin and rennin. Pepsin breaks down proteins into much smaller units that can be more easily processed in the small intestine. Another function of the gastric juices is to destroy any potential microbiological invaders.

When incoming food mixes with the gastric juices, a semi-fluid mass called chyme is formed. The pH of the chyme must reach a certain level of acidity before signals are sent to allow the pyloric sphincter, or valve, to open naturally and pass the chyme into the small intestine. If the stomach acid is too weak, the correct pH level cannot be reached and this process cannot take place. In this case, it is the weight of the mass in the stomach that triggers this valve to open. The chyme, including all unwanted bacteria and parasites, is then pushed with the help of the peristalsis, a wave-like muscle contraction, into the small intestine for the next stage of digestion.

Symptoms of weak stomach acid - hypochlorhydria - include bloating, belching, diarrhea, hair loss, weak fingernails, heartburn, stomach upset, and undigested food in the stool. The most common cause of this condition is aging, stress, alcohol consumption, medications, zinc deficiency and bacterial infections. There is also a link between hypochlorhydria and diseases such as allergies, anemia, asthma, autoimmune diseases, and skin problems such as acne and psoriasis.

The *H. pylori* bacterium may be one of the survivors of hypochlorhydria. It is usually harmless, but sometimes it weakens the stomach's natural defenses and can attack its lining and cause ulcers. Diagnosis of this infection can be made by stool antigen test, polymerase chain reaction (PCR) test, breath test and endoscopic biopsy. Other low acid survivors can include parasites. Some live in harmonious coexistence with the human body, but others are troublesome and may cause digestive issues. In the past, it was not easy to detect them, but today's sensitive PCR test gives reliable results. Every living being – including parasites, bacteria and viruses – contains the unique genetic material (DNA) of its species. PCR testing amplifies even the smallest DNA material and compares it with existing data, which leads to a high success rate in diagnosis. Gastrointestinal experts recommend treating infections or parasites first before proceeding with other treatments as this can prevent recurrence of diseases.

If you have a problem with low stomach acidity your healthcare provider may add a betaine hydrochloride (betaine HCL) supplement to your protocol to ensure proper digestion and absorption of nutrients. For some people, the betaine HCL works great; for others, it can be painful or even ineffective. Finding the right dose requires an experienced healthcare provider, as it depends on several factors, such as age and overall health. Taking this supplement on suspicion can be counterproductive. In some cases, it can even increase intestinal gas production. As the name implies, hydrochloric acid is a mineral acid that contains hydrogen. People with methane dominated gas production may also be affected because one methane molecule is formed from four hydrogen atoms. A gentle alternative to betaine HCL is half a teaspoon of apple cider vinegar in a small amount of water five minutes before each meal, or some bitters as directed by your naturopath or nutritionist.

The Heidelberg Test for Stomach Acid can provide clarity about whether you have problems with stomach acidity. This test involves taking a baking soda solution and swallowing a small electronic device the size of a vitamin capsule that measures the pH level of the stomach. Although this test is not cheap, it can detect diseases such as hypochlorhydria, hyperchlorhydria, or achlorhydria. A home version of this test, although not very accurate, is to mix ¼ teaspoon of baking soda in around 5 ounces (150 ml) of cold water. Take this solution first thing in the morning before you eat or drink anything. Measure how long it takes for the first proper belch to occur. If you have not belched within 3 to 5 minutes, you may have low stomach acid. If you belch immediately, you could have too much of it. However, this test is only a rough indicator, and you might like to do the Heidelberg Test for Stomach Acid to rule out any serious issues.

Please note that a regular use of non-steroidal anti-inflammatory drugs (NSAID) such as aspirin and ibuprofen in combination with a betaine HCL supplement can damage the gastrointestinal mucosa and increase the risk of stomach ulcers.

---

I came across this home stomach acid test with baking soda very early in my health journey. At the time I didn't even know there was such a thing as low stomach acid, which made me curious and I tried this test to it. In the morning, I prepared my baking soda and drank the solution. I waited and waited – nothing happened. After half an hour there was not even the slightest burp. That was enough to make me think something was terribly wrong with my stomach acid. During my SIBO treatments, I repeated the test a few times, and fortunately the expected burping did not fail.

# LIVER

One of the functions of the liver is to protect the body from harmful substances, viruses, bacteria, fungi and parasites. Through our environment, we are exposed to many toxins. Every time we eat, drink, or apply something to our skin, the liver tries to filter and eliminate any harmful chemicals. The liver is also busy breaking down excess hormones and old blood cells, storing vitamins and minerals, metabolizing carbohydrates, fats, and proteins. As if that were not enough, the liver also regulates the amount of circulating cholesterol. This process is important for the health of the immune and digestive systems. Another well-known task is its production of bile. This dark green to yellowish-brown fluid consists of water, salts, cholesterol, and the pigment bilirubin. It emulsifies foods such as fats and proteins into tiny droplets, helping to speed up the digestive process. The liver has a sophisticated network of bile ducts so that this fluid can be transported within the organ and to the gallbladder, where it is stored for later use.

Although the liver is a resilient organ, it does not always find it easy to do its job as we often treat it badly. Alcohol, cigarettes, fatty foods, some herbs, supplements such as vitamin A, medications, and contraceptives that contain high doses of estrogen or progesterone, are among the many substances that can damage this organ. There are many facets of liver disease that can lead to liver cancer or dysfunction, regardless of culture, age, or gender. Dr. Patricia Lalor from the University of Birmingham UK says: "Liver disease kills more people than diabetes and road accidents combined". Liver cancer is the second leading cause of death worldwide.

If you have complaints like bloating and pain in the upper abdomen, they may be related to the liver, for example, due to a simple cyst. Liver cysts are fluid-filled cavities that can be congenital or caused by parasites (*Echinococcus*). They do not grow quickly and are usually not a cause for concern. Most often they are discovered in adulthood via a scan. More serious liver diseases include fatty liver disease (alcohol and non-alcohol versions), liver scars (cirrhosis), Type 2 diabetes, cystic fibrosis, hemochromatosis (an overload of iron) and hepatitis.

We cannot live without the liver, and it is important that we take care of it and not overload it with harmful substances. This organ is quite undemanding, but we need to get out of its way so that it can do its job. A better lifestyle is a good start and can be achieved through a healthy, nutrient-dense, low-sodium diet, moderate alcohol consumption, and not smoking. Healthy body weight and regular exercise are not only good for the immune system, but also for the liver. Avoid the use of recreational drugs and practice safe sex, as this will protect you and your partner from hepatitis B and C. Vaccination for hepatitis can save lives.

In Traditional Chinese Medicine (TCM) emotions and physical health are closely linked, and the liver is associated with anger, stress, stagnation, frustration, bitterness, and resentment. These emotions can get out of hand and create an imbalance in the body, especially when they occur suddenly and last for a long time. Be mindful if you feel constantly stressed and upset, as this can affect the function of this organ.

One might think that everything is fine with the liver, as nothing is felt. Surprisingly, while looking for something else, a specialist discovered an irregularity in my liver. The herpetologist advised me to discontinue with the progesterone cream (a natural hormone replacement) I was using because it can affect the liver, which I did. This situation has prompted me to have a closer look at my everyday habits that could potentially harm this organ over time. Certain ingredients in cosmetics, plastic utensils with soft grip handles that release BPA or other harmful chemicals, alcohol consumption, or simply heating food in a plastic container in the microwave can be the cause.

## GALLBLADDER

The gallbladder is a small sac underneath the liver. This sac acts as a reservoir in which the bile becomes more concentrated and saltier. This modified bile has alkaline properties and helps provide the best environment for digestive enzymes. When bile is needed, a gentle muscle contraction pushes it out of the gallbladder into the pancreatic duct, and finally into the small intestine, where it is used in the digestive process.

You've probably heard of gallstones before. These are crystallizations of bile. Most of them are harmless, but sometimes they can block one of the bile ducts. This life-threatening condition can lead to liver damage or inflammation of the pancreas. Scientists know that gallstones develop through an imbalance of bile components, but they are uncertain why this happens. One reason could be that the gallbladder does not get emptied entirely or regularly enough. If the gallbladder doesn't perform well, fat-soluble vitamins like A, D, E, K1, and K2 cannot be adequately absorbed. These vitamins are essential for proper growth and development in children as well as for the digestive health of us all.

Under certain health circumstances, it is necessary to remove the gallbladder (cholecystectomy), which means that the interim storage for bile is no longer available. Bile salt will drip continuously into the small intestine. At first, this may not seem like much of a worry, but people can suffer afterwards from bile reflux, which can cause inflammation of the stomach lining. A study found that there is a higher risk of developing SIBO after cholecystectomy. Interestingly, when you have SIBO, without any interventions, it can cause the same problems as a cholecystectomy. In this case, bacteria can change the bile mixture so the body is no longer able to absorb fat or fat-soluble nutrients. This can lead to nutrient deficiency and malabsorption. A sign of the latter can be steatorrhea. Scientists associate a higher mortality rate with cardiovascular disease related to increased malnutrition. If you cannot produce enough bile yourself, there are ways to support your gallbladder with supplements that contain ox bile or bile salts. Talk to your healthcare provider if you may need it.

In people with celiac disease, an immune reaction occurs in which antibodies are formed against gluten found in grains such as wheat, rye, and barley. This reaction can damage the intestinal lining and promote inflammation. The cells in the gastrointestinal mucosa usually send information to other organs to participate in the process of digestion. They tell the liver to produce bile and the pancreas to produce enzymes and when to release them. However, if these cells are absent or damaged, the natural communication system is disrupted, and the gallbladder may malfunction or become inflamed. People with celiac disease are at risk of gallbladder failure and releasing toxins into the body, leading to an emergency.

To prevent gallbladder disease, maintain a healthy weight and exercise regularly and moderately. Avoid crash diets or very low-calorie diets as this releases additional cholesterol from the liver and produces more bile, which may hinder a proper emptying of the gallbladder.

My stool was big and bulky, at the same time hard to flush. Really annoying! This bulkiness occurs because a high proportion of fat and gas are not well processed and can be an indicator for steatorrhea. I never thought to tell my doctor about it, but when I did, his eyes suddenly widened because it was another clue to my health. Not every floating stool is a sign of a serious disease, but it should be a cause for concern, especially if it is clay-colored and sticky. In my case, it was an indicator for celiac disease. As soon as I went on a strict gluten-free diet, my stool started to normalize and became more substantial and darker.

## PANCREAS

The pancreas is a vital organ located in the upper-left abdomen behind the stomach. This organ has two primary biological functions. One is to build the hormone insulin, which is released into the bloodstream to regulate blood sugar (glucose) levels. Diabetes occurs when the pancreas cannot produce enough insulin, or develops a resistance to it. In either case, cells in the pancreas try to produce more insulin to manage blood glucose levels. In this process, cells wear themselves out or are destroyed. Another function of the pancreas is the production of enzymes that help to break down carbohydrates, proteins, and fats into small molecules. These enzymes are activated when they meet the juices of the small intestine. A lack of stomach acid can be the cause of a decrease in pancreatic enzymes and bile production. The consequences of this condition can result in steatorrhea. Exocrine pancreatic insufficiency is the name for deficiency of digestive enzymes.

Some people are born with cystic fibrosis, a pancreatic disease that produces an abnormal quantity of thick and sticky mucus within the body. These thick secretions host bacteria that can severely affect the lungs, pancreas, liver, kidneys, and gut. Alcohol consumption is the main cause of pancreatic damage. Interestingly, celiac disease has a similar effect on the pancreas as alcohol, putting people with this disease at increased risk of developing pancreatitis. A damaged pancreas can lead to diabetes and promote pancreatic cancer. This type of cancer is aggressive and has a poor survival rate. Sometimes there is a tiny possibility of living without the pancreas, but the price is a lifetime of insulin injections and digestive enzyme pills, among other limitations. I can't stress enough how important it is to see a doctor if you have floating stools or signs of pancreatitis such as pain, malabsorption, weight loss, or diabetes. There is a reason for these symptoms, and it must be addressed as soon as possible.

## SMALL INTESTINE

Now we come to the small intestine, which can cause us so much trouble. This organ is divided into three sections: the duodenum, jejunum, and ileum. It is as thick as a middle finger and the length from 10 to 20 feet long (3 to 6 meters). There are not many microbes in the first part of the small intestine, but this situation changes towards the end of this organ, closer to the large intestine. The small intestine primarily absorbs nutrients. With the help of the pancreas, gallbladder and liver, it continues the digestion process.

The semi-solid chyme from the stomach is gradually released into the small intestine. This process can take up to one to two hours, depending on what has been eaten. This slow process is important because it maximizes the absorption of nutrients into the body. When the chyme arrives in the small intestine, it moves onto a velvet-like surface. If you look through a microscope, you'll see that there are finger-like projections - known as villi - on the surface of the small intestine. If you get even closer than that, you'll see that each villus has cells on its surface that also have finger-like projections called microvilli. Together they provide a huge surface area for the absorption of nutrients.

Any microorganisms that were able to pass through the stomach unhindered find a cozy home in the small intestine and multiply. This new population creates a bottleneck situation in this organ, as its abundance restricts the pathway for incoming food. Some of these residents metabolize bile salts and insoluble components, which can lead to fat malabsorption or diarrhea. Others, such as *Klebsiella* species produce toxins that damage the mucosa, impair absorption functions, and create secretions that mimic tropical sprue. The microorganisms feed on carbohydrates and create gases that lead to the typical SIBO and IBS symptoms. A small amount of gas can be absorbed through the wall of the small intestine and enter the bloodstream, and the rest of the gas is usually trapped in the intestine and expands the organ.

Any undigested food particles that reach the small intestine extract water from the body by osmotic effect, leading to bloating, pain, and discomfort. Considering this, it's no wonder we might look like we're in the second trimester of pregnancy! Under these circumstances, pressure is exerted on the mucosa of the small intestine, to such an extent that it can form microscopic holes. The undigested food particles can enter the bloodstream through these openings. This condition is known as leaky gut. The immune system recognizes these particles as foreign invaders and activates antibodies to fight them. Food sensitivity and inflammation as well as autoimmune diseases can develop. I will discuss the topic of leaky gut in more detail in a later chapter.

## MIGRATING MOTOR COMPLEX

Have you ever wondered why you can sometimes hear a rumbling noise in your tummy after you have eaten? It is a rhythmic, wave-like movement of the stomach and small intestine that attempts to clean up after a meal, called the MMC. It ensures that any remaining food, bacteria and yeasts are moved along to the large intestine. This movement is not the same as peristaltic waves already mentioned. The main feature of the MMC is that it works between meals and stops working when new food comes along. Researchers believe that the MMC is controlled by the hormones motilin and ghrelin. It seems that the autonomic nerves - especially the vagus nerve - also play an important role in its function, especially within the stomach.

If you are the type of person who likes snacking all day long, your MMC can't do a good job. Imagine there is a nonstop party at your house! The peristalsis is responsible for moving the celebrating crowd along to the after-party, whereas the MMC tries to clean up after the last guest has left. If new guests arrive before the MMC has finished its work the situation can get out of hand. The MMC tries to tidy up the intestine, around six times per day. It doesn't matter if you are awake or asleep. Food, medication, or stress can interrupt the "housekeeping" tasks of the MMC. The same applies to gum chewing. Dr. Pimentel says that the stimulation in the oral cavity signals the body to produce gastric acid and get into eating mode. This trigger can be enough to stop the MMC. For many people, a dysfunctional MMC is one reason why they developed SIBO or IBS in the first place.

If you want to help the MMC do its job, allow enough time between meals and drinks. After food enters the body, the MMC needs around two hours before it can begin its work, and almost another two hours to complete it. Fast for at least four hours, if not five hours, between meals. If you follow this rhythm, you can have up to 4 meals a day. Please don't consider this way of eating if you're underweight, as it may physically harm you. Talk to your healthcare provider if you feel unsure.

The consumption of pure water, or plain, unsweetened tea or coffee does not interrupt the MMC. Adding milk or sugar to these drinks will halt the MMC. Dietary supplements are also considered as food because they contain all kinds of fillers, such as lactose. The consumption of a small amount of fat or acidic liquids is tolerated without disturbing the process of the MMC. For fats, this could be a spoonful of coconut oil, olive oil or some ghee, and the acidic liquid could be a little bit of apple cider vinegar or a squeeze of lemon or lime juice in some water.

Eating every 4-5 hours became second nature to me. While getting used to this rhythm, I noticed how often I wanted to put something in my mouth unnecessarily. To overcome my cravings for sweets, I developed a new habit: sipping on warm water during the day. It calms my nervous system, feels good in my gut and counteracts dehydration. It's worth trying – just put some hot water into a thermos, maybe add a small slice of fresh ginger or lemon, and you're good to go. If you prefer a more stylish option than a thermos, you can buy a double-walled glass flask with a stainless-steel infuser that will look great on your work desk.

A prokinetic agent supports the MMC by strengthening and stimulating it without disturbing its natural rhythm. There are several naturopathic and pharmaceutical products available, each having benefits and drawbacks. Talk to your healthcare provider about what is best for you. Sometimes it may be necessary to take more than one type of prokinetic. Experts recommend taking prokinetics for at least six months, especially after an antimicrobial treatment. Don't be fooled if your symptoms have completely disappeared for a while. Keeping things moving is one of the key factors in avoiding a recurrence of conditions like SIBO and IBS.

## ILEOCECAL VALVE

The ileocecal valve (ICV) is a sphincter valve that separates the small intestine from the large intestine. It is located in the lower right part of the abdomen, near the appendix. This valve works like a trap door that opens and closes periodically to let chyme move through the digestive tract. It is supported by hormones and nerves. During the phase of absorption of nutrients, vitamins, and minerals in the small intestine the ICV remains closed. Once this work is done the ICV opens to allow the chyme to move forward into the large intestine. Ideally, the ileocecal valve then closes again quickly to prevent the chyme from slipping back into the small intestine.

A dysfunction of the ICV can lead to SIBO, IBS and other gastro-intestinal problems. The valve can be chronically closed, resulting in a backlog of content in which bacteria can easily multiply in the small intestine. The valve can be permanently open, causing reflux from the large intestine into the small intestine, including all the microbes that don't belong there. Causes of dysfunction include surgical intervention, joint misalignment, rough foods, inadequate nerve supply, nutrient deficiency, appendectomy, and scar tissues. One study found that children with an anatomic alteration such as short bowel syndrome are more susceptible to SIBO, as quite a few of these children have a dysfunctional ICV or even no ICV at all.

Symptoms of ICV syndrome may include a feeling of tightness in the lower abdomen, abdominal pain, constipation, diarrhea, malabsorption, nausea, and shoulder pain. Tunnel syndrome and inflammatory conditions such as arthritis are also associated with this syndrome. If you are planning a colonoscopy, you can ask the gastroenterologist to check whether the ICV is closed or open. This information may help you to determine if you have a problem with it. To counteract an impaired ICV, you can perform a maneuver at home to improve its function. Dr. Jacobi demonstrates this three-minute ICV maneuver in a YouTube video (see resources). She recommends doing it daily for at least two weeks to help to improve symptoms.

## LARGE INTESTINE

We come to the last stage of digestion, which takes place in the large intestine, which is 5 feet long (1.5 m) and 2.5 inches thick (around 6.5 cm). The term colon is a generic term commonly used to describe the large intestine and its component parts - the cecum, appendix, colon, rectum, and anus.

When the chyme leaves the small intestine it first passes through the cecum, where the previously unabsorbed fluids and salts are further absorbed and mixed with mucus. As waste products continue to move through all parts of the colon, it is lubricated, residual fluids and salts are absorbed, and fecal matter is stored until rectal nerves tell the brain to open the anus and let it go.

The rectum runs through the pelvic floor and is consequently in close connection with it. This muscle group holds organs such as the bladder, intestine, uterus and prostate. Normally, it is firm and thick and helps to prevent accidental urination or defecation. Sometimes these muscles can weaken, stretch, or become too tight. Causes include age, pregnancy, child delivery, systemic diseases, bad posture, chronic constipation, obesity, smoking, and menopause. Research has shown that women are more prone to pelvic floor problems such as organ prolapse and stress urinary incontinence, which is urine leakage when coughing, sneezing, laughing or running. Pelvic floor dysfunction affects not only women, but also many men. Both men and women can experience anal incontinence, the urge to go to the bathroom more often than necessary, constipation, bloating, lack of sensation or pain during intercourse.

Fortunately, it is possible to control and treat this condition. There are surgical and non-surgical alternatives. The latter can include medications, pelvic floor exercises, biofeedback treatments, and relaxation techniques. You can seek help from a physical therapist who specializes in this topic. They will assess your pelvic floor function and create an exercise program tailored to you. Some healthcare providers are trained in visceral manipulation devised by Jean Paul Barral, an osteopath and physical therapist from France. This gentle manual therapy is applied to the internal organs and works especially well for bladder disorders. If you cannot find a visceral manipulation therapist, you can consult an osteopath who may be able to help you. Correct body alignment is a key to overcoming this problem.

## MICROBIOME

The gastrointestinal tract contains one trillion microbes and an average of 160 different bacterial species. Most of them cavort in the large intestine. Over the past decade, science has worked hard to understand the composition of this microbiome. Today, we know that its inhabitants play an important role in our health. For example, they synthesize micronutrients such as vitamin K, B12, biotin, folic acid, and pantothenic acid (vitamin B5), and support the absorption of calcium, magnesium, and iron. They also collaborate with the immune system, and together they fight off invasive microorganisms.

Our first contact with these microbes occurs during birth, followed by breastfeeding and direct environment, which provides us with a variety of beneficial microbes. Unfortunately, a healthy microbiome can be compromised by bacterial infections, antibiotic treatments, medical procedures, poor diet and unhealthy lifestyle. When the microbiome is compromised, it may take some time to transform it into a diverse and healthy one again. It is not as responsive as you might think - changing it is like turning a cruise ship around. After diet and lifestyle changes are made, it can take up to thirty days to see improvements. For some people it may take months or even years. So don't get frustrated if you don't see results right away. Look at your current situation as an opportunity to change your lifestyle and become healthier. It's up to you to make these changes. Your healthcare provider can assist with their knowledge, but ultimately it comes down to you and your daily choices.

# CONCEPT SUMMARY

» Our gastrointestinal system is a collection of specialized organs. A dysfunction in one of these organs may not be compensated by another. This system is not autonomous, as it interacts with other parts of the body such as the brain, immune and nervous systems.

» The gut analyzes everything we put in our mouth or on our skin. It passes this information on to the brain, which has to decide how to deal with these substances.

» The sophisticated communication between the gut and the brain (also known as the gut-brain axis) uses the vagus nerve to transmit information. If the vagus nerve is impaired or damaged, the gut-brain relationship may be disrupted, leading to misinformation and thus to health problems.

» Digestion begins with the first sight and smell of food and ends with the excretion of waste products; in between, almost the entire body is involved. During fasting, the MMC is still operating, transporting undigested materials to the exit; it stops working as soon as eating is resumed. A dysfunctional MMS can lead to an overgrowth of bacteria in the small intestine.

» Impaired gastrointestinal motility results in either too much or too little water being absorbed in the digestive process and can affect the intestinal mucosa. The result is either diarrhea or constipation.

» Each person has a unique microbiome that harbors trillions of microorganisms, including thousands of different species of bacteria, fungi, archaea, and viruses. Sometimes this ecosystem can get out of balance and compromise health.

# STRESS

Humans are complex beings who live in a multidimensional environment. Everything around us and within us influences us, and also affects our digestive system. That's why it is not enough to hope for a magic pill to cure your gut problems. Rather, you need to look at yourself holistically and explore the obstacles that stand in the way of your healing process. This may include removing possible toxins from your environment, as well as addressing psychological issues that may have arisen from small and large traumas in your past. It is hard, if not impossible, to find a healthcare provider who can guide you through all the hurdles and requirements to help you overcome your intestinal issues. You will probably have to build your own team to support you in various ways. This may include a healthcare provider who gives you a broader overview of your problem, while other specialists may give you a deeper insight into specific areas of concern. There are also many alternative services that can help you adopt a new lifestyle. If you are lucky, all these people will work together to help you; if not, you'll have to be your own health manager. But let's start with the topic of stress, because its influence on the gastrointestinal system should not be underestimated.

Stress is not to be confused with busyness. It is about how the body reacts to internal or external pressure and tension. It has many origins and can manifest in various ways, whether it is physical, psychological or both. Each person reacts to stress differently. In the same situation, one person can feel tension and another not. There are different types of stress. Physical stress can arise from the perception of danger, while anxiety triggers emotional stress. Noise and crowds can cause environmental stress. And then there's chronic stress, the feeling of being constantly overwhelmed, which can lead to fatigue and withdrawal from social interactions. Often, it is a mixture of all these factors that can cause health problems.

When we experience a stressful situation, for instance something alarming we see or hear, signals are sent to the brain to evaluate the incoming information and determine the appropriate action. The body has a mediator that is responsible for transmitting this information. This is where the autonomic nervous system comes into play – a jack-of-all-trades, it acts as a regulator, activator, coordinator, and communicator. The regulator's job is to minimize harm to the body but maximize its function. When we experience a short-term imbalance, the activator tries to overcome the challenges by mobilizing physical resources. The coordinator manages the continuous flow of information in all directions, so that it is available for the control center – the brain – and the rest of the body. The communicator has a special function, as it is responsible for our appearance and makes it easier for others to read and assess our state of mind. Are we friendly or threatening? Are we sociable, or do we want to be left alone? Are we in pain or do we feel pleasure?

In order to respond appropriately, the autonomic nervous system is always busy monitoring and assessing our external environment and regulating our internal environment. It is not surprising that inaccuracies in the transmission of information within the body can lead to incorrect decisions that may affect health and wellbeing. To understand why we respond to our environment and stressful situations in one way and not another, it is worthwhile learning about the autonomic nervous system, which tries to fulfil the body's need for balance.

Our body's nervous system is made up of billions of nerve cells that are responsible for everything we do. It contains two main systems: the central nervous system, which includes the brain and the spinal cord, and the peripheral nervous system that controls all other nerves in the body. Within the peripheral nervous system lies the autonomic nervous system, which controls organs and glands, regulates bodily homeostasis including heart rate, blood pressure, respiration, digestion, and sexual arousal. This system consists of elements of the brainstem, some spinal nerves, and cranial nerves. The vagus nerve is the longest and most complex of all cranial nerves and is responsible for both sensory activities and body movements.

The autonomic nervous system has changed during evolution to ensure survival through adaptive and flexible strategies. Within this system there are three subsystems: the enteric, sympathetic, and para-sympathetic nervous systems. The enteric nervous system is embedded in the lining of the gastrointestinal system and controls motility, secretion, and all local and physiological requirements such as blood flow. It is also in a two-way communication with the central nervous system and receives input from the sympathetic and parasympathetic nervous systems via the vagus nerve. An interesting feature of the enteric nervous system is that it can function independently from the brain and spinal cord and is also referred to as the "second brain". Nevertheless, the enteric nervous system is still a mystery, so further research is needed to get a more accurate picture of its nature.

During my research, I came across some exciting information about the enteric nervous system that I'd like to share with you. One study highlighted that a functioning enteric nervous system at birth is critical to enable oral food intake. A dysfunction in this system can lead to inadequate motility, which can contribute to the development of gas-trointestinal diseases such IBS and chronic constipation, even in later years. In children, this condition can also have lasting effects on their neurological development. In addition, a study on animals points out that neonatal stress, such as a separation from the mother, can cause long-term health problems. This experience can be the cause of visceral hypersensitivity later in life. In general, all of us, adults, and children alike, are susceptible to changes in the gastrointestinal system, which then affects the enteric cells (neurons). A common intestinal infection alone can trigger a process that promotes diseases like IBS, long after the infection is gone.

There is evidence that IBS may be related to serotonin. Serotonin is a hormone that has many roles, one of which is a neurotransmitter (chemical messenger) that sends signals to the enteric nervous system. Serotonin not only influences our sleep and mood, but also has a major impact on pain perception and intestinal function. The culprit could be a malfunction of the serotonin transmitter, a protein that helps to remove this hormone from the gut. Intestinal bacteria are the main producers of serotonin as they supply 95% of the body's needs and release it into the intestinal lining. If this hormone hangs around in the gut for too long, symptoms such as cramps, pain and diarrhea may occur. The discovery of the link between serotonin levels and IBS in recent years opens up new therapeutic possibilities, as drugs can block or stimulate serotonin receptors to reduce abnormal bowel activity.

Let's take a closer look at the other two subsystems of the autonomic nervous system: the sympathetic and parasympathetic nervous system. Traditionally, these two systems are often seen as competing, as the sympathetic nervous system provides the "fight-or-flight" response, and the parasympathetic nervous system provides the "rest and digest" response. But is it true that they are in opposition? Dr. Stephen W. Porges, a scientist and professor of psychiatry, has introduced a new perspective on this topic with his Polyvagal Theory. He says that all subsystems of the autonomous systems should be considered hierarchical and not as opposing, since they are nested within each other. From an evolutionary perspective, the youngest of these subsystems are recruited first when the body is in need. If necessary, the older ones come into play later. Dr. Porges notes that our most modern development is the ventral vagal nerve circuit in the parasympathetic branch. Then comes the sympathetic nervous system, and finally the ancient dorsal vagal nerve circuit, which is also found in the parasympathetic branch. All of these systems operate independently of each other.

The parasympathetic nervous system generally support immobilization, which is normally associated with relaxation, growth, and recovery.

In this state, the ventral vagal nerve circuit triggers feelings of peace, security, and social engagement. It slows the heart rate, relaxes muscles and increases bowel activities. This nerve pathway also controls the facial and head muscles, which supports variations in facial and vocal expression for social interactions. When this pathway is activated, our middle-ear muscles are more activated, making it easier to recognize other human voices. We are better at making eye contact to foster bonding with others. Dr. Porges says in this state we literally show our heart on our face. This ventral nerve circuit can even downregulate or restore the sympathetic defense system, whichever is appropriate. We can make a positive contribution to the activation of this nerve circuit by engaging with each other in a social and purposeful way.

In contrast, the sympathetic nervous system is mobilized in emergencies and dangerous situations. It can make us alert and confident. When this system is activated, muscles tense, blood flow is stimulated, especially for lymphoid organs, and the body releases a large amount of the stress hormone cortisol. In exchange for this hormone production, the body reduces other important functions such as those of the immune system. Dr. Porges says, in this state, the body is mainly focused on being alert, and we are not particularly sociable or empathetic. If a person in this state tries to engage with others, they are more likely to get into an argument. Nowadays, it is common for many people to get caught up in the sympathetic response for too long. This is not without risk, as it can lead to chronic stress which in turn leads to adrenal fatigue or burnout.

Have you ever noticed that when your gastrointestinal symptoms worsen you tend to provoke those around you? I have. It seems that my underlying health issues trigger the sympathetic nervous system response and I fall into the trap of attacking, blaming, or judging others. It is so important to notice in time when I have physical discomfort. Then I'd better withdraw for a while, even if it's just to the bathroom for a few minutes. This way, I can give myself enough time to process my discomfort and feelings.

According to Dr. Porges' Polyvagal Theory, the last of the three nerve circuits is the ancient dorsal nerve pathway that is integrated in the parasympathetic branch. It normally supports us when we feel safe, but it also intervenes in traumatic or dangerous situations. In such situations, a reflexive biological reaction manifests itself by putting us into a state of immobilization, like a "freeze" – a behavioral shutdown or even a collapse. In this state, the body saves metabolic resources and lowers the heart rate. A similar effect can be observed in reptiles when they feign death in response to perceived danger. Since these animals require little oxygen for their small brains, it does not harm them to shut down their body system for a certain period of time. However, humans have a higher oxygen demand, and it may be difficult to return to normal after such a traumatic event. Gastrointestinal problems, hearing hypersensitivity, poor vocal intonation and diminished facial expression are common after-effects. The severity of these symptoms depends on how involved the individual's nervous circuit is during the event. You may not be aware that you have been in such a "freeze" situation because it happened in your childhood – during abuse or birth trauma. Whereas as an adult, the feeling of being completely numb and distanced from oneself is more real, especially in situations of sexual or physical abuse. After such a terrible event, you may blame yourself for not fighting or running away. Dr. Porges emphasizes that it is important to understand the survival techniques of the body and its instincts so that this negative thinking can be avoided. Instead of feeling guilty, it is helpful to praise your body for what it has done for you and for making it through this situation alive.

Each of these nervous system circuits has its own duty of care in the body. The ventral vagal nerve circuit of the parasympathetic nervous system is responsible for the regulation of all organs *above* the dia-phragm. In contrast, the dorsal vagal nerve circuit controls all organs *below* the diaphragm. Operating predominantly under the influence of only one nervous system circuit may negatively affect the corresponding organ.

Stanley Rosenberg, an American-born, Denmark based body therapist and close friend of Dr. Porges, created a beautiful metaphor in his book *Accessing the Healing Power of the Vagus Nerve. Self-Help Exercises for Anxiety, Depression, Trauma, And Autism*. He says that the three circuits of the autonomic nervous system, as mentioned in the Polyvagal Theory, are like Goldilocks and the three bears. When Goldilocks was walking through the woods and entered the house of the three bears, she found three bowls of porridge on the table. One was too hot to eat, the other was too cold, and the third was just right. After she ate, she looked for a bed, as she felt very tired. The first bed was too hard, the second too soft, but the third was just right. Rosenberg compares Goldilocks' experiences to the quality of muscle tone in the three nervous system circuits mentioned above.

The muscle tone is the tension in a muscle at rest. It maintains posture and stabilizes joints during sudden changes. Low muscle tone describes floppy and weak muscles. The clinical description is hypotonia. While increased muscle tone makes it difficult for the body to move normally and to flex. The extreme form is spasticity. When the sympathetic nervous system is activated, it creates a too hard or too hot muscle tone, and the activated dorsal vagal branch of the parasympathetic nervous system can create a too soft or too cold muscle tone. The ventral vagal branch, with its qualities of social commitment and sense of security, creates a muscle tone that is just right. The body can be manipulated using body therapy or exercises to bring it into this healthy state. In his book, Rosenberg offers simple physical exercises that can easily be integrated into everyday life.

Since the vagus nerve has a close relationship with the autonomic nervous system, especially the parasympathetic nervous system, modern science pays a lot of attention to this cranial nerve in order to understand diseases and general health. The vagus nerve originates from the medulla of the brainstem, meanders down the sides of the neck, through the chest, and is connected to many muscles and organs, such as the heart, respiratory and digestive organs, on its way to the rectum. Eighty percent of its fibers are responsible for sensory, taste, visceral and somatic information. The remaining 20% of its fibers control the motility of the gastrointestinal tract, heart rate, and anti-inflammatory pathways. One of its main tasks is to sense information about the state of the internal organs and transmit it to the brain. This role makes it an important participant in the two-way communication between the brain and the gastrointestinal tract; the so-called "gut-brain" axis. The vagus nerve influences emotional and cognitive functions, and states such as mood and anxiety. Nowadays, it is recognized that not all mental disorders have their origin in psychology, they can also be of physical origin.

When the vagus nerve receives signals of inflammation in the body, it alerts the brain and simultaneously activates anti-inflammatory resources (neurotransmitters) to regulate the body's immune responses. An impairment of this nerve is associated with many diseases. For example, people with inflammatory bowel disease often suffer from a mixture of autonomic nervous system and psychological disorders. Ulcerative colitis is related to vagal dysfunction, while people with Crohn's disease may have an issue with the sympathetic nervous system.

A pilot study presented at the Annual European Congress of Rheumatology (2019) suggested that stimulation of the vagus nerve could be a novel approach to treating rheumatoid arthritis. In this study, fourteen participants who did not respond well to medication were implanted with a miniature neurostimulator called "MicroRegulator", resulting in a significant reduction in symptoms. This treatment was well tolerated by all participants.

These examples are not the only interesting areas of study concerning the vagus nerve. There is also its relationship with the heartbeat. The more active the vagus nerve is, the lower the heart rate (of course, within a healthy range) and the more variable the time between the individual heart pulses. A method known as heart rate variability (HRV) measures the time between beats. This test can be done in a laboratory environment or with less sophisticated equipment at home, using devices such as an Oura Ring, CorSense from Elite HRV or Inner Balance from HeartMath. Some scientific theories emphasize that a higher HRV leads to increased stress resilience, better cognitive performance, social functioning, and better energy regulation. At the same time, it promotes emotional balance so that we can experience positive emotions, appreciation, courage, and love. Dr. Navaz Habib, a functional medical practitioner, speaker, and author of the book *Activate Your Vagus Nerve. Unleash Your Body's Natural Ability to Heal* explains that HRV can give us higher levels of fitness, cardiovascular health, and longevity. In contrast, an impaired HRV performance can lead to emotions such as frustration, anxiety, worry, and irritation. It can also affect food intake and weight gain.

There are various practices and exercises that can increase the vagal tone and stimulate the vagus nerve. Dr. Habib advocates that the first and most effective way is to breathe properly. Learning a deep breathing technique and practicing it, especially before meals, does not just calm the nervous system, but also improves digestion. He says that the easiest way to activate and heal a loss of vagus nerve tone is to regularly expose yourself to a cold shower for a short time. In his book, he describes other techniques such as humming, singing, laughing, and gargling to release muscle tension – for example, in the larynx – to stimulate the motor fibers of the vagus nerve. Sleeping on the side is preferred, as this keeps the airways free at night and improves the HRV levels. Listening to music or music therapy are also great tools.

Dr. Porges and his colleagues have spent the last twenty years developing the Safe and Sound Protocol (SSP), a therapeutic listening program that targets the vagus nerve using modified music. Based on the Polyvagal Theory, this intervention trains the middle ear muscles to better perceive human voices and the emotional meaning of speech.

An early version of this intervention is known as the Listening Project Protocol, which first received attention in the field of autism spectrum disorder. The SSP is designed to reduce stress and auditory sensitivity while improving social engagement and resilience. It helps to restore a sense of safety and calmness in the autonomic nervous system.

Researchers discovered that inattention and stressors that interfere with social engagement, as well as auditory sensitivity, anxiety, and trauma-related conditions, can be improved in a relatively short period of time through the use of SSP. There is a five-day program for children and adults that can help one become more regulated, focused, and engaged. This program involves listening to modified music for one hour per day on consecutive days. It can also be used in 30-minute segments. However, some people may need to repeat the whole program a few of times before they achieve the desired result. If you are interested in SSP, contact a healthcare provider, educator, medical professional, or psychologist who is trained in this protocol. They can support you and provide the necessary equipment and modified music. Some therapists like to use this intervention at the beginning of their counseling sessions to help their clients achieve a calmer physical and emotional state for improving communication.

Other ways to calm the autonomic nervous system and the vagus nerve include stimulation with pharmacological medications, tube feeding (enteral nutrition), complementary medicines such as acupuncture, and physical exercise. Some researchers advocate techniques such as autogenic training, meditation, deep abdominal breathing, repetitive prayers, hypnosis, biofeedback, cognitive and relaxation therapies, qi gong, tai chi and yoga - including laughter yoga. One study shows that yoga is a safe and effective method for patients with ulcerative colitis. Practicing yoga ninety minutes per week, over a minimum period of nine weeks, resulted to significant improvement in the participants' quality of life. All these practices and methods have one thing in common: they not only have a positive effect on the vagus nerve, but also release the hormone oxytocin, which builds confidence and promotes positive emotional and social well-being.

Let me introduce you to autogenic training, which is a method that was developed in the 1920s by J.H. Schulz, Germany. It is well studied for its positive effects on anxiety disorders, mild-to-moderate depression, functional sleep disorders, headaches, migraines, hypertension, coronary heart disease, bronchial asthma, somatoform pain disorder, and Raynaud's disease. Some people use it to manage pain or to prevent chronic stress. You can learn it through self-study or take a course that runs weekly, usually eight to ten weeks. This technique involves performing specific exercises for a few minutes, several times a day. By teaching the body to respond to verbal commands, it helps to control breathing, blood pressure, heartbeat, and body temperature. You experience a state of physical relaxation and a peaceful mind. It is important to practice this technique regularly, as it takes a few months to master all the exercises. As a result, you will have a tool that you can use at any time for the rest of your life. A word of caution applies to people with diabetes or heart disease because this technique may raise blood pressure. If you have one of these conditions, you may want to learn autogenic training under medical supervision.

There are many different forms of meditation with different origins, techniques, and approaches. Thanks to this diversity, it is possible for anyone to learn and perform meditation – whether sitting, lying, or even in motion. Often the trickiest part is finding the right meditation for you that fits your current mental and physical state. If you have never meditated before, a good place to start is using a free mobile phone meditation application like Smiling Mind or Headspace. They offer guided meditation for every level of experience. Alternatively, you can try one of the meditations offered by Deepak Chopra, a physician, Ayurveda advocate, author, and founder of the Chopra Center for Wellbeing. Or choose one of the many resources and inspirations from the publishing house Sounds True.

If sitting on a chair or floor is not your cup of tea, consider a walking meditation as taught by the Vietnamese Buddhist monk and Zen master Thich Nhat Hanh. He was a spiritual leader, poet and peace activist who reaches thousands of people with his simple mindfulness teachings. You can still learn the art of mindful living in short and long-term stays in one of his monastic practice centers located around the world such as the Plum Village monastery in southwest France. He has also written many books that may inspire you to incorporate mindfulness into your daily life to reduce stress and support your ventral vagus nerve and parasympathetic nervous system.

When you are connected to your heart, life seems so much less stressful and problems appear in a more positive light. We have all experienced the difference between feelings of separation from ourselves and others, and feelings of harmony and compassion. The key has always been the heart. When we love, trust grows. A troubled heart, on the other hand, can lead to anxiety, worry, irritation, and frustration. Dr. Rollin McCraty of the HeartMath Institute explains that the heart has its own nervous system that sends more information to the brain than vice versa. This means that the heart strongly influences our thinking, reactions, and self-regulations. Since 1991, the non-profit HeartMath Institute has dedicated its research and information to connecting and harmonizing the heart and the mind. Their goal is to help people live more fulfilling lives. Much of their research focuses on reducing and preventing stress. Their website has a wealth of information and is worth checking out.

There are many practices such as yoga, deep breathing, visualization, and mantras to connect the heart and mind, and learn loving kindness. One of them is the Meditation on Twin Hearts by Master Choa Kok Sui who is originally from the Philippines. He developed the Modern Pranic Healing system that uses energy to support the healing of the physical body, mind, and soul. In some traditions, this energy is called prana, chi, ki, mana, pneuma, ruah, or even vital energy and life force.

Pranic Healing is a no-touch modality that can be easily learned and applied for the benefit of others and yourself. The Meditation on Twin Hearts is a central element of the work. When practiced regularly, it can improve mental concentration, physical and mental health, and may bring harmony into your life. To learn this meditation, you can attend a free meditation evening or an online event from one of the many Pranic Healing centers around the world. Check out the website of the Institute for Inner Studies, to find the closest center to you. You may also like to buy one of Master Choa Kok Sui's books or CDs for self-study.

Meditation, prayer, mindfulness, and gratitude practices are all wonderful tools to calm the mind and to be more resilient to stress. A regular relaxation and meditation practice lowers blood pressure, slows the heart rate and supports the digestive and immune systems. Be mindful, trying to relax and have a "must do" attitude is counter-productive. It is best to find something you like to do on a regular basis, even if you just take the time to look out of the window for a while and think about nothing.

I would be lying if I said that it was easy to incorporate meditation into my daily life. Over many years, I made various attempts to experience the benefits of meditation. I tried several approaches, coming from different religious backgrounds. My best effort was a ten-day Vipassana meditation retreat. This meditation technique was rediscovered by Buddha more than 2500 years ago and is still taught today. I prepared myself with smaller retreats before plunging into the ten days. Such a long retreat is a serious undertaking, as one is deeply confronted with oneself. Today, I regularly practice various meditation techniques, such as Master Choa Kok Sui's Meditation on Twin Hearts, because I no longer want to miss the peace and clear mind that such a practice gives me.

## MENTAL STRESS

Humans have a deep-rooted need for social interactions to feel safe, connected, and valuable. We spend our whole lives trying to satisfy this need, though there are times when we feel especially disconnected and lonely. Regardless of culture, age and socialization, social disconnection and loneliness can affect both physical and mental health. It is not easy to meet our need for social interaction in this day and age. An increasing number of people have difficulty navigating through this rapidly changing world with its new, intangible virtual connections. Dr. Lise Van Susteren, an American psychiatrist, and her co-author Stacey Colino describe in their book, *Emotional Inflammation. Discover Your Triggers and Reclaim Your Equilibrium During Anxious Times*, how modern life creates symptoms that are comparable to post-traumatic stress disorder (PTSD), causing intense feelings of anxiety, helplessness, depression, and restlessness. These emotions overlap with our personal everyday challenges and contribute even more to our stress. Concerns for the future affect everyone. The authors say: "… if you don't think you're experiencing emotional inflammation, you're probably not paying enough attention to how you're feeling".

The authors mention that the more sensitive the nervous system becomes, the more disproportionate reactions to new and negative influences, such as bad news, become. When we are exposed to acute and/or chronic stress, the prefrontal cortex, the large front part of the brain that controls thoughts, actions, and emotions, changes in structure – it shrinks. The amygdala, a small almond-shaped grey mass in the brain that controls aggression and is responsible for the perception of emotions, such as anger, fear, and sadness – expands. A week of stress, or even a single event, can trigger this process. Looking at the big picture of society and the environmental challenges of today, the deleterious effects on the prefrontal cortex is probably quite common. Poor cognitive skills and susceptibility to stress are well known and are likely to become more evident in future generations.

It is important to understand how and why our physical and mental health is affected by certain lifestyle choices. To ground ourselves again, the authors suggest spending time in nature and regaining our natural rhythm by not messing with our biological clock, for example, getting enough sleep. Changing negative thinking patterns and learning critical thinking to filter information more efficiently is another step toward wellbeing. One recommendation that was unexpected for me was that one should develop a tolerance for discomfort, which is not the same as ignoring feelings, or warning signals from the body. I think they got to the heart of the matter. It is common for people to dislike being confronted with inconvenience or discomfort. For most, it is torture to endure a slight pain or discomfort. They look for a solution in the form of supplements, medications or other "miracle cures". Since this approach doesn't really work, Dr. Van Susteren and Ms. Colino encourage practicing mindfulness by accepting feelings and reactions instead of fighting frustration, anxiety, and anger. By "letting go" of these feelings, an inner space is created in which clearer choices can be made. Feelings and emotions are contagious and can influence your environment in any direction. If you put forth the courage and effort to learn about yourself, the people around you can change as well. You will be surprised how quickly this can happen and situations will change for the better instead of constantly deteriorating.

There are thousands of different approaches to improve mental health, and it is often not easy to find the right one when you need it most. If you have a chronic physical health problem, you can tell your doctor that you want to add a mental health plan to your medical treatment. They may be able to recommend a counselor or therapy to you. Another approach is to select from among the many alternative therapies. The choice is too wide and would go beyond the scope of this book to list them all. But if you venture out into this world, try to find a trustworthy and professional practitioner to avoid disappointment and charlatanism. At the same time, keep an open mind. The following are some of the methods I encountered on my road to recovery. They have helped me and could possibly help you too.

First, there is hypnotherapy, which uses hypnosis to connect with your subconscious mind to bring about healing. This complementary therapy is carried out under the guidance of a certified therapist or medical professional, who puts you in a relaxed state – a type of trance – to make you more receptive to therapeutic transformation. Researchers at Monash University in Australia, led by Dr. Simone Peters, have found a 70-80% reduction in gastrointestinal symptoms in IBS when gut-related hypnotherapy was undertaken. This therapy can promote better communication between the brain and the gut, so that information is more easily transmitted and retrieved in both directions. Hypnotherapy is like a guided meditation, with the goal of seeing yourself through a heightened state of consciousness and correcting unhealthy behavior patterns. There is a misconception that once you are under hypnosis, you no longer have free will or control over your mind. This is not true, because you are always able to bring yourself out of this relaxed state at any time. Perhaps you remember the last time you had a daydream or listened to music intensely. It only takes a little distraction to get you out of that "zone" and back into everyday life. The same applies to hypnosis. You do not need to prepare for a session. Wear comfortable clothes and make sure you are well-rested, otherwise you might fall asleep during hypnosis. Unlike self-treatment where you listen to a hypnosis CD at home, a trained therapist can take an individualized approach to your health concerns and mental state. They will be available to talk with you before and after treatment to discuss any findings or questions. Hypnosis may not be appropriate for people with severe mental illness.

I really enjoyed hypnotherapy because it helped me to relax and overcome some hidden negative beliefs I had about myself. My therapist made special recordings for me, which was great as I could deepen my practice in the comfort of my own home. It was especially useful when I suffered from severe bloating. Then I withdrew from the world for a short time and turned to her voice. It was amazing how quickly my body responded and recovered. I can't say that hypnotherapy helped me get rid of all my gastrointestinal problems, but attending these sessions was an important step in making me feel more comfortable in my body.

Since the key to healing is to release hidden stress, tension, and trauma in the body and mind, there is no way around practicing deep relaxation and self-enquiry to achieve positive long-term results. When you have cast off mental baggage it is much easier to meet yourself and others. There is a part of us that never changes, that is always in the present moment and at peace. If we enter this space regularly through meditation, we are able to recall this experience in our daily lives.

iRest® (Integrative Restoration), is another method that can help you to overcome mental obstacles. It was developed over the past forty-five years by Dr. Richard Miller, a clinical psychologist, researcher, author, spiritual teacher, and yoga scholar. He combined the traditional yoga nidra practice with western psychology and neuroscience. It is a guided mindfulness meditation that fosters a deep relaxation through breathing, body awareness and guided imagery. Studies show that this program can help to reduce depression, anxiety, insomnia, and chronic pain, and enhance resiliency and wellbeing. iRest has been successfully used with soldiers returning from Iraq and Afghanistan who suffered from PTSD. As a result, it is often taught around active duty and veterans' military environments, homeless shelters, prisons, hospices, seniors' facilities, universities, clinics, as well as in yoga and meditation studios worldwide. Anyone can learn and use this method, regardless of their physical ability or previous experience with meditation. iRest can be learnt in a group setting with a trained instructor, or in a self-directed program by using audio. For the latter, you can download free audio files from the iRest website, or purchase a CD from the publisher Sounds True. iRest is usually practiced lying on a soft mat to keep you comfortable for about forty-five minutes. The instructor or audio will guide you through the ten levels of the program. In the first sessions, you will learn to connect with your heart, formulate an intention and find an inner place where you feel completely secure. This special inner place can be revisited at any time during the practice or in your daily life. It provides a safe haven when you feel overwhelmed by emotions, thoughts, or other life circumstances. You then learn to observe what is happening in your body. Are there tensions, shallow breathing, feelings, and emotions that want to come up? By witnessing your thoughts without judgment, you can see the beliefs you have about yourself. The program works with opposing viewpoints to help you accept all experiences as they are. This practice can lead to joy, wellbeing and bliss that comes from your heart and spreads throughout your body. These feelings can dissolve into an awareness of the "Self" – the peaceful, untouchable being within you I have mentioned earlier. At the end of the exercises, you reflect and try to integrate your experiences into your everyday life. The advantage of learning this technique with a certified instructor is that they introduce you to the program step by step, and support you when needed. Once the method is learnt, it is a tool for life.

Recently, I visited a Core Energetics body psychotherapist to address a physical issue. To my astonishment, just one session brought about a profound shift in my mindset and significant relief from my symptoms. This system has a long history dating back to the 1940s, when Dr. John Pierrakos and Dr. Alexander Lowen were clients and students of Wilhelm Reich. They were also influenced by Carl G. Jung. Both became physicians and psychotherapists in the U.S., where they developed Bioenergetics, a psychotherapy practice that takes a body-oriented approach. They experimented with exercises and postures to release chronic muscular tensions, repressed emotions, and restricted breathing. By working on the breathing, they were able to create an energetic connection between the mind, heart, and genitals to heal their clients on different levels. In later work, Dr. Lowen emphasized his work on the release of anger, while Dr. Pierrakos increasingly pursued spiritual concerns in his work. Due to their different approaches and interests, they separated in the 1970s. Through personal influences, Dr. Pierrakos refined and renamed Bioenergetics to Core Energetics, still a body-oriented psychotherapy, but with the focus that each person has the innate capacity for love and healing that can be unlocked through this system. Core Energetics includes somatic psychological principles based on the concept that humans experience their environment not only through their thoughts and emotions but also through their body. The program works in four stages: Letting go of old beliefs that no longer serve a useful purpose; working on destructive aspects of our personality; grounding and centering; and finding life purpose. A Core Energetics practitioner must go through several years of training before they are allowed to offer their service. A consultation normally involves some counseling and bodywork – this could be breathing exercises, specific movements, vocal expressions, self-massage, or with consent, a therapeutic gentle touch. A session can take place in person or via video conference, with individual or couples' sessions, or group seminars. This is a gentle approach to achieve long-term, sustainable results to overcome negative and sabotage patterns.

Emotional Freedom Technique (EFT), also known as tapping, could be another tool of choice to overcome negative beliefs, patterns, and emotions. This technique was developed in the late 1990s by Gary Craig and emerged from the Thought Field Therapy of Roger Callahan, a U.S. clinical psychologist. EFT is a self-help method that is easy to learn. By stimulating acupuncture points in a certain order, combined with the verbalization of psychological statements, it can bring emotional relief and reduce stress. Even though this technique sounds a bit voodoo, many studies have researched EFT. For example, a review paper by Dr. David Feinstein examined around fifty studies that met his evidence criteria. He concluded that a tapping technique, when used properly, can lead to a positive change in a person's neurochemistry and release emotional pain associated with traumatic memories. You can learn this technique in seminars, online classes, or find a therapist who can guide you through the process and provide psychological support.

Kinesiology is a form of therapy in which the reaction of a muscle to certain statements or questions is observed. This technique was developed in the 1960s by Dr. George Goodheart, who combined his knowledge of the meridians used in TCM with other therapies. He recognized that meridians and organs are connected to certain muscles, mirroring the physical and psychological processes in a person. In 1964, Dr. Goodheart developed a simple test method that works without equipment: the muscle test of applied kinesiology was born. Since then, kinesiology has undergone several ground-breaking developments and is still taught and applied today. One of the modern directions is neuroenergetic kinesiology developed by Hugo Tobar. His method works directly with the nervous system and takes into account additional energetic structures and imbalances. Kinesiology is based on the principle that the human body has an innate healing energy that will always do its best to take care of the body. The treatment bypasses the conscious mind and establishes a direct communication with the subconscious, and thus with the body. The client is asked to hold a body part, for example an arm or a leg, against a gentle pressure applied by the practitioner. The muscle's reaction is translated into an answer related to the subject being explored. There is no reliance on a verbal response from the client. Conclusions are drawn about possible energy blockages or influences to which the client is currently exposed. Kinesiology seeks to identify and correct the causes of imbalance so that blockages and stress can be removed. The practitioner will ask the body what needs to be done to support its healing abilities. Sometimes a specific movement pattern must be practiced, or the answer lies in dietary changes, physical exercise, letting go of emotion, rebuilding energy, or even addressing spiritual concerns. Professional kinesiology practitioners have undergone years of training to learn how to assess and rebalance the body.

> I had the good fortune to live with an excellent kinesiologist for several years and served as his test subject during his training. It is incredible how many fears and stressors I was able to leave behind during that time. It also was a joy to see him working with children because they really blossomed through this gentle method, and conditions like chronic bedwetting or behavioral problems became a thing of the past. When you find the right practitioner, they can work wonders.

Paying attention to your diet could be another approach to dealing with mental health problems such as anxiety and depression. Some foods can ease or worsen these conditions because they affect the biochemistry and hormones in the body. On the other hand, the right nutrients can help correct dysfunctions and imbalances. There are two great books on this topic that I came across. The first is *The Anti-Anxiety Food Solution. How the Food You Eat Can Help You Calm Your Anxious Mind, Improve Your Mood and End Cravings* by Trudy Scott. The title says it all, doesn't it? She addresses the problem by explaining in detail how biochemistry is involved in these conditions, and ways to counteract them. She also gives tips on how to improve digestion. It is most informative, but it is not a recipe book. The second book is *The Happy Kitchen. Good Mood Food* by Rachel Kelly and nutritional therapist Alice Macintosh. They offer great recipes and back them up with background information. The authors are passionate about helping others overcome the burden of anxiety and other mental health issues.

# DIETARY STRESS

Having a healthy nervous system does not mean that the system always remains calm. We are confronted with too many different situations in the course of our lives for that to be true. The more flexible and resilient the nervous system is, the more it helps us stay mentally and physically healthy. The opposite is true when we are out of balance and have too much stress. Unless stress is managed, whether it is of a psychological and/or physical nature, your health may not improve. It might be pointless to impose a treatment regime that focuses mainly on diets and supplements if stress plays a huge part in your life.

For many of us, food gives us pleasure and an emotional connection to our social environment. We enjoy catching up with friends over a meal or having a vibrant family gathering. Without food, it's half the fun. Sometimes the taste, smell and texture of food can catapult us back into the past, especially into our childhood. Good and bad memories may then guide our food choices. There are days when food makes us happy and satisfied. On others, negative experiences and stressful situations spoil our appetite and may cause us to overeat and gain weight. We may then question our body image and self-esteem. The constant confrontation and oversaturation of information about food and nutrition in the media is not exactly helpful either. There are so many fixations on magical "superfoods", and many so-called experts claiming to know the right way to eat – it's no wonder we are confused, vulnerable and don't know what to eat anymore. The nervous system responds to these stresses and signals the digestive system that it is drawing resources away from it to cope with these "emergencies". If your digestion is not already compromised, the response to them could be the tipping point.

With a compromised digestive system, many consider certain foods to be of particular concern and begin to omit them, in the hope that this will be the way out of their misery. But with this practice, a creeping fear slowly makes itself felt - perhaps other foods should perhaps also disappear from the plate. The downward spiral continues, taking with it anxiety and worry, which in turn affect digestion. Eating, drinking, and oxygen are the main players in the metabolic process, but they are not the only things that influence this process. Everything we experience, dream, feel and think contributes to a great extent. Marc David says in his book *The Slow Down Diet. Eating for Pleasure, Energy and Weight Loss*: "Metabolic power is not only about what we eat but who we are when we're eating. And it's not merely about how many calories you burn but how inspired you are in life". He is the founder of the Institute of Eating Psychology, a teacher, speaker, and author. In the last four decades, he has accumulated a wealth of knowledge regarding nutrients, psychology and eating. His clinical experience and research show that eating disorders, obesity, and digestive problems have their origins primarily in physiological stress and the hectic pace of daily life. He says that negative thoughts about food and one's life directly affect the nervous system and accompanying hormones, and the way we digest food. He also stresses that countless hidden mantras like "fat makes me fat," "I am not loveable unless I have a perfect body," "I am a victim," "I have to try harder to get healthy," "I need to find the perfect diet to be happy," "there's not enough time to nourish me," "I feel guilty eating," "I have to eat this way because others know better," and many more, are a sources of judgment, punishment, self-abuse, shame, and guilt only add further stress to our lives.

Mr. David further points to the dilemma of dividing food into "good and bad" categories. If one has eaten a "bad" food, perhaps because no other was available at the time, a resistance arises in the body that impairs digestion. If you have eaten it on purpose, you may feel guilty afterwards because you think you shouldn't have. If your goal is to eat only "good" foods, then you are unnecessarily discriminating and limiting yourself. It can lead to the belief that you are better than others because you know what is good, or on the contrary, you are not worthy of enjoying the fullness of life. The question is, who actually defines good and bad food? Depending on each person's perspective, culture, and lifestyle, one and the same food can have different values. Realistically, I can only agree with Marc David who says "food is morally neutral. So is every other object in the universe".

If you suffer from SIBO or IBS, you may be advised to follow a special diet to alleviate symptoms. I'm not saying that you shouldn't do this as it may give the relief you need. Yet, such diets can also cause emotional stress – as they can clash with your cultural and ethical eating habits, and force you to learn new cooking skills, eat separate meals at the family table, and limit your social interactions as some dietary requirements can make it difficult to attend special events and travel. All of this can leave you feeling overwhelmed, lonely, and helpless. An expectation that a diet will cure you can even lead to frustration, especially if the desired result is not achieved or a relapse of the disease occurs.

> You may have already read between the lines; I have a somewhat ambivalent relationship with these elimination diets. I had never dieted in my life before I was diagnosed with SIBO and IBS. I seriously believed that these diseases can be cured by diet. The diet gave me only short-term relief, but still the price was high. On top of my daily efforts to cook for the family, I had to prepare separate meals for myself. When I went out to eat, I always had to be on my toes and check the ingredients. On these occasions, people usually engaged with me about their food issues, because this topic seems to preoccupy so many people. This intense preoccupation with food began to stress me out. I love food, but I don't want to think and talk about it all the time.

Anxious or obsessive behavior when planning and preparing a meal is another stressor. There is even a disorder that results from an obsessive fixation on healthy eating - orthorexia nervosa. The general question is – what is more harmful, the food or the stress, or both together? The focus should clearly be on reducing stress at all levels and creating more peace for the mind and body. To achieve this goal, take it one step at a time as you make a switch to a new diet. Do not put too much pressure on yourself. You will make mistakes, as I did, but you will slowly learn what is right for you, and what is not. Even then, nothing is set in stone. As your health improves, you may be able to introduce foods you never imagined eating, or you may no longer enjoy some foods. When you eat, how often you eat, and the environment in which you eat is as important as what you eat. Taking your meals in a calm atmosphere can make a huge difference to your gut.

The pleasure and curiosity of learning something new can be a healthier approach. Open yourself up to these experiences and start to nourish yourself. To do this, you need to stop thinking of food as an enemy and welcome it into your life – perhaps not from fast-food chains! The way we normally eat is just a perception of our mind and society. Imagine you are born into a culture with completely different eating habits; perhaps you wouldn't question eating a snack of grilled grasshoppers. Just because you have eaten a particular way for a long time doesn't mean it's right for you now.

If you start a special diet because of your health condition, it doesn't mean you have to follow it for the rest of your life. It is meant to help relieve your symptoms by giving your body a break from the foods it struggles with, but it is not a permanent solution. Of course, it's desirable to cure SIBO, IBS and other gastrointestinal diseases as soon as possible, but it's equally important to be sensible. This health journey is about getting to know your body and adopting a new lifestyle, and not stressing on what you can or can't eat anymore.

A key experience for me was at a breakfast buffet in an airport hotel in Korea. On one side of the buffet was offered a typical western breakfast with jam and toast, bacon and eggs. On the other side there was a traditional Korean breakfast with many ingredients unknown to me. Interestingly, overweight people were more likely to choose the western breakfast, while visitors with a slim appearance preferred the other side. It's incredible how we are conditioned. Fortunately, with a little awareness, we can change our eating habits.

# EXERCISE

Regular exercise has many health benefits, for example, it helps with weight loss, reduces the risk of heart diseases, and strengthens bones and muscles. It can increase serotonin levels and contribute to better sleep. It can be lots of fun and sociable. Most people benefit from it, regardless of age, gender, or physical ability. However, exercising is easier said than done when you suffer from gastrointestinal problems. Depending on the severity of the condition, it may be difficult or even impossible to perform. Some people experience symptoms such as nausea, heartburn, urinating problems, diarrhea or even bleeding, so it is not surprising that physical activities are avoided.

Even if it's challenging for you to overcome physical discomfort and pain, it's worth doing. It comes down to finding the right balance and figuring out what type of exercise suits your condition. Research has shown that physical activity significantly improves IBS symptoms, has a protective effect on the gut mucosa and promotes bile production in the liver. Exercises strengthen the abdominal muscles and stimulate intestinal motility. With this in mind, there is every reason to exercise regularly.

Not all exercises are equally good for the digestive system. In fact, it is not uncommon for endurance athletes to experience gastrointestinal problems because the intense training can lead to physical stress. When the body is challenged in this way, it requires more energy to transport oxygen and nutrients to the muscles and to regulate the body temperature through the skin. Meanwhile, other parts of the body - including the digestive system, may have up to 80% less blood flow, slowing down their functions. With decreased blood flow, sphincter activity and transit times are out of rhythm, which in turn affects the MMC. An insufficient fluid intake will worsen symptoms. There are some things to avoid to prevent any further gut issues such as bending over and drinking water from a bottle while cycling which can put too much strain on the stomach, or eating just before or straight after exercise, because digestion can be disrupted. This is especially true for when you eat foods that are difficult to digest, such as protein, fat, or fructose. With a little care you can benefit from moderate to light exercise because it's fantastic for physical and mental health, especially for digestive system performance. Keep your gut happy and stay well hydrated.

I haven't exercised for many years because I was too busy to fit it into my daily routine. Then came severe back pain, I felt sluggish and stiff. I knew I had to do something if I wanted to get healthy, but it wasn't until an osteopath recommended Pilates that I signed up for a class. Thanks to his treatments and regular classes, I no longer have back pain. To this day, I do Pilates to strengthen my core and back muscles, which is such an important foundation for other sports. My current Pilates instructor is very diligent about executing the poses correctly, as the deep muscle groups need to be engaged. I prefer his approach compared to my experience in a gym. There, the exercises were performed so quickly that it was impossible to follow the trainer, let alone perform them properly. Besides the Pilates classes, I try to do some physical movement every day. It's like "snacking". It could be a short workout such as a quick jump on the cross trainer, some weight training, a brisk walk in the park or on the beach, or just the 5 Tibetan Rites after meditation. Going hiking with friends and family on the weekend is another great way to socialize and be active.

# SLEEP

Alongside nutrition and exercise, sleep is the third pillar of wellbeing. For one third of our lives we are in this passive state. Even though we do not consciously experience ourselves in sleep, the body uses this time productively. During sleep, the body and mind recharge, leaving us alert and refreshed when we wake up. The body tries to restore and repair tissues, save energy, and strengthen the immune system. At the same time, the brain works on long-term memory and integrates new information. Every time we rest, the entire machinery for maintaining the body is in full swing.

When our sleep is constantly interrupted it can't do this job. Imagine trying to focus on your daily work and being constantly pulled out of it. It can be a pretty annoying situation. At the end of the day, you might think "what did I actually do today?" and hope tomorrow will be a better day with more satisfactory results. Our body is in a similar situation. If its work is disturbed at night because we constantly wake up, it cannot perform quality maintenance. The result can be a series of physical and psychological health issues, including anxiety and depression.

How much sleep you need depends on your age, lifestyle, and health. In general, most adults need an average of eight hours of sleep to feel fresh and rested the next day. It's probably a good idea to match your lifestyle to your sleep needs, rather than the other way around. It's simple math – if you have to get up at 6 a.m., you should go to bed by 10 p.m. to get enough sleep.

Before my diagnosis of IBS and SIBO, I was a bit of a night owl. I really enjoyed the quiet hours after the kids went to bed. That was my "me time". My usual bedtime was 11pm, sometimes even later. I often didn't feel refreshed the next morning, but I would pull myself through the day and be tired again by mid-afternoon. In the course of treating my gastrointestinal disorders, I changed my habits and now go to bed at 10 pm, which has made a huge difference. If I haven't found time to meditate during the day, I do a little breathing exercise by Dr. Andrew Weil before I close my eyes. It helps me fall asleep faster.

Most living things, including animals, plants, and microbes, follow a biological rhythm (the circadian rhythm) that runs on a 24-hour cycle. During this time, our eyes sense changes in the environment and send signals to the brain to adjust body functions to the given conditions, for example, to make us more tired or awake. This circadian rhythm not only controls sleep and wakefulness but also our appetite, body temperature, blood pressure, and hormone levels. It is a creature of habit that functions best within a set routine. Yet, this rhythm can be disrupted by exposure to light at unusual times, altered sleep patterns, temperature, physical activity, social interaction, and unusual mealtimes.

The hormone melatonin plays a key role in the proper functioning of the circadian system. Its production is stimulated and slowly released into the bloodstream when it gets dark, which is usually at sunset. This is the time when the body needs to wind down, expecting sleep two hours later. Melatonin levels peak when it is completely dark and usually remain active for around twelve hours until daybreak. Our habits of staying up late and being exposed to bright light suppresses the production of this hormone. Modern devices play a key role in this situation, keeping us awake by providing us with an available activity, but these devices are not the only culprits. Actually, all lights at night-time disturb the sleep process, especially lights in the blue and green spectrum. For a healthy sleep, it is therefore advisable to stop looking at electronic devices two hours before bedtime. Since this is difficult to accomplish for most of us, an alternative would be to look at red spectrum light as it has the least effect on the melatonin production. Free software applications for electronic devices and computers, like f.lux or Redshift help with weary eyes and promote better sleep. They automatically adjust the color-temperature on your screen to the time of day. Manufacturers like Apple offer a built-in system to change the color-temperature of the screen by activating the "night-shift function". Of course, it is harder to implement a light strategy when you are a shift worker. In this situation, try special glasses that block out the blue color spectrum. You can balance your evening activity by trying to expose yourself to plenty of natural bright light during the day. Although light has the greatest influence on the circadian rhythm and melatonin, it may be worth making dietary changes to counteract sleep problems. Melatonin, like the hormone serotonin, depends on the availability of tryptophan, an essential amino acid that the body cannot synthesize and must obtain from food. It is commonly found in both plant- and animal based proteins.

Studies have shown a lack of sleep leads to increased levels of inflammation and white blood cell counts, even in healthy young people. The immune system is weakened when sleeping habits are geared towards late nights and early mornings. Cytokine, whose molecules stimulate the body's cells to communicate with each other, is an important indicator that the immune system may not fully recover from sleep loss. There are two types of cytokines: one is a pro-inflammatory that can worsen disease, and the other is an anti-inflammatory, which promotes healing. Sleep deprivation increases pro-inflammatory cytokines and thus has a negative effect on cells. Researchers found that just one night of insufficient sleep can reduce insulin resistance and that chronic sleep deprivation can lead to obesity.

I know what you're thinking, no more staying up late or even partying. What a dull life. But remember: if you want to get healthy, you need to support your body. It needs enough sleep to recover and do its work at night. During the healing process, you may feel the need to sleep more than the recommended eight hours. Don't worry – it's perfectly normal. Let your body guide you, it will tell you what it needs. Later in your recovery, you may sleep less, but for now, be sure to have a regular, early bedtime.

There are many reasons why people cannot sleep deeply even though they wish they could. Insomnia is a sleep disorder that makes it difficult for people to fall asleep, stay asleep, or return to sleep after waking up at night. Typically, one does not feel well-rested and suffers from lack of energy the next day. This can lead to irritability, or even progress into depression or mood swings. Older people, shift workers and women are more prone to this condition. The latter group may go through several stages in their lives where sleep becomes a problem, such as pregnancy, infant care and menopause.

Trudy Scott, a certified nutritionist, author, lecturer, and founder of the nutrition practice, Every Woman over 29, explains in an interview with Misty Williams at Your Best Sleep Ever! Summit 2020, that insomnia can have many causes, such as low gamma-aminobutyric acid (GABA), low serotonin (a pre-cursor of melatonin), low blood sugar levels, and high cortisol levels. Parasites are another possible cause of waking up at night and not being able to go back to sleep. Ms. Scott says symptoms of low GABA is often associated with physical tension, such as tightness in the shoulders, intestines, and abdomen. It can also result in unwanted thoughts and a busy mind that keeps you from falling asleep. The classical signs of serotonin deficiency include irritability, anger, bad mood, winter blues, perfectionism, negative self-talk, imposter syndrome, and cravings in the afternoon and evening, often satisfied with sugar or carbohydrates.

Many people try to relax and get a good night's sleep by drinking alcohol in the evening. Ms. Scott explains this form of self-medication is counterproductive and can damage the intestinal mucosa leading to leaky gut syndrome. The result is deficiency in zinc, vitamin B6 and magnesium, which is needed to make proper neurotransmitters. She adds that prescription medications containing benzodiazepines such as Ativan, Valium and Xanax should only be used in acute situations and for a short period of time, as they can be addictive and lose their effect after some time. Instead, her treatment approach is to take amino acids, for example GABA or theanine for GABA deficiency, and tryptophan/5-HTP for serotonin deficiency. These supplements provide immediate symptom relief and each addresses the individual underlying problem.

Another cause of insomnia may be diet. Sugar, for example, allows gut bacteria to throw a party. One of these partygoers is the *Costridium* bacterium, which can cause diarrhea and affect sleep quality. Interestingly, one study found that women with chronic fatigue syndrome have more *Clostridium* bacteria in their gut that may influence their hormones. The connection between the gut and the brain is not to be underestimated. What is fed to the gut affects the brain and vice versa.

For more information on sleep or implementing healthy sleeping habits visit the Sleep Health Foundation or the National Sleep Foundation. There is also the streaming service Brain.fm, which has developed music that interacts with brainwaves – that is, small electrical currents that flow between the brain's neurons – to promote better sleep, focus on work, and relaxation. Their science-based approach is to alter these brainwaves through computer-generated music (bimodal tones). You may need to listen to the music regularly before you experience a positive effect. Remember, sleep is one of the best remedies we have – allow yourself more of it rather than less.

Besides caring for children, entering menopause was another phase in my life where getting enough sleep was a challenge. Before going to bed, I worried about whether I would sleep through the night, which didn't help either. One day I was visiting one of those craft markets. While browsing, I came across a stall selling traditional Ayurvedic massage oils. My eyes lingered on a sign that read "Ksheerabala oil: nourish and nurture. Helps insomnia and menopausal symptoms". At the sight of this big promise, I was curious and bought it. And yes, it really helps me – I rub a small amount on my feet and temples twenty minutes before bed. It puts me in a state of relaxation so that I can fall asleep more easily. These days I wake up refreshed, often even a little earlier than necessary – extra time for a quiet cup of tea before the busy day starts.

# CONCEPT SUMMARY

» In today's world, it is common to live in a permanent spiral of stress, which can be of physical or psychological origin. In this state, the enteric nervous system and the sympathetic nervous system are on heightened alert, triggering the fight-or-flight response, which can lead to impairment of some bodily functions, including those of the gastrointestinal system.

» The autonomic nervous system consists of three main nerve circuits. In the parasympathetic branch is the ventral vagal nerve circuit, which provides the "rest and digest" response and controls all organs above the diaphragm. The ancient dorsal nerve circuit, also part of the parasympathetic nervous system, can put us in an immobilization or "freeze" mode, this nerve path is responsible for the organs below the diaphragm. The third nerve circuit is the sympathetic nervous system, which is responsible for the "fight-or-flight" response that is activated in certain situations such as danger or stress.

» The vagus nerve oversees a variety of important bodily systems, such as the anti-inflammatory pathways, and is the main component of the parasympathetic nervous system. To maintain long-term health, it is necessary to support this system and its ventral vagal nerve circuit, the "rest and digest" response. Regular use of stress management methods are recommended for this purpose.

» Move your body regularly to support your digestion, but do not overdo it by training for a marathon. Make sure you are well hydrated.

» Sleep is one of the most important remedies we have and should be given special attention. The body and mind need this restful time to maintain and regenerate. You can support this effort by creating good sleeping habits by putting your devices in a red-light spectrum in the evening and allowing two hours screen-free time before bed.

# INFLAMMATION

When parts of the body become inflamed, there is usually redness, swelling, heat, and sometimes pain and physical impairment. Inflammation protects the body from infection and kills pathogens. It initiates a repair process in the tissues and provides stability for damaged areas. Let's assume you have a wound: your immune system will trigger proteins called cytokines which then send signals throughout the body to take further action. It's like calling the ambulance, and a doctor arrives with a bag full of white blood cells, hormones, and nutrients to solve the problem. To take advantage of these substances, the blood vessels become more permeable so that a swarm of white blood cells can target the injured area and begin removing foreign bodies, germs, and dead or damaged cells. Almost simultaneously, the body sends fluid to the damaged area to remove waste. This process can cause swelling and pressure on nerve endings, leading to pain. Hormones help to clot the blood, heal damaged tissue, and are responsible for any fever. We have all experienced this type of acute inflammation – with a cut, sore throat, sprained ankle, or acute bronchitis. It usually lasts only a short time, and the body quickly heals itself. However, when inflammation becomes a long-term condition, things are different because chronic inflammation is more persistent and can sometimes last a lifetime.

In chronic diseases, a distinction must be made between low-grade and high-grade inflammation. The latter is more obvious as it occurs in diabetes, celiac disease, rheumatoid arthritis, and inflammatory bowel diseases. Low-grade inflammation is often overlooked for years. It silently causes problems and increases the risk of developing autoimmune diseases, cancer, cardiovascular problems, insulin resistance, type 2 diabetes, and neurodegenerative diseases such as Parkinson's and Alzheimer's. There are various reasons why these low-grade inflammatory processes are activated. The most common causes are microbial infections from viruses, bacteria, parasites, and fungi, burns and frost-bite. Irritants such as radiation, chemicals, diesel exhaust particles, ozone, and endotoxins in the water can also contribute to this situation. When you add to this mix a lack of nutrients and oxygen, which leads to insufficient blood flow and tissue death, it is no wonder that health problems tend to escalate.

There are several tests to detect inflammation and infections in the body. The Serum Protein Electrophoresis, Erythrocyte Sedimentation Rate, C-Reactive Protein, and Plasma Viscosity blood tests are commonly used to identify the increase in proteins in the blood. Your doctor may also check for ferritin levels. Ferritin is an iron-storing protein that is usually screened when iron deficiency is suspected. Based on the test result, the doctor can distinguish between iron-deficiency anemia and anemia due to chronic inflammation. It is common in SIBO and IBS that iron levels - and vitamin B12 - are low, because bacteria love to feed on them. High ferritin levels can be an indicator that excess iron has accumulated in the liver, heart, and pancreas, which can lead to life-threatening diseases such as diabetes, and failure of these organs. In any case, you should have your iron levels checked.

It is not easy to reduce inflammation. Diet could be a part of the solution. There are foods that promote this condition, while others prevent or even mitigate it. The Mediterranean style diet is of particular benefit here, as it contains many anti-inflammatory foods and limits pro-inflammatory foods such as red meat and refined carbohydrates. This diet is rich in antioxidants, fiber and healthy fats.

# MICROPLASTIC

The human body is not spared from the plastic pollution that we have inflicted on the planet in the last seventy years. Plastic permeates our everyday lives, and it is impossible to imagine life without it. It is a versatile, inexpensive, and practical material. Since the 1950s, we created about 8.3 billion metric tons of plastic that have ended up in landfill, which is more than the weight of one billion elephants. Its popularity is still growing, as we produce around 320 million tons annually, 40% of which is used for disposable packaging. Most of this plastic waste is not biodegradable and takes hundreds or even thousands of years to decompose, if at all. It is more likely that it breaks down into smaller particles, especially when exposed to ultraviolet (UV) light and abrasion. These particles are from between five millimeters to one-thousandth of a millimeter in size and are referred to as microplastic. Plastic particles below this size are called nanoplastics and are not visible to the naked eye. The abrasion of vehicle tires on road surfaces creates nanoparticles, and this is one of the main sources of environmental pollution. Nanoparticles can easily be inhaled or washed into waterways.

There are countless ways in which plastic enters our environment. We have now introduced plastic particles into virtually every ecosystem on this planet. It is therefore not surprising that scientists at the Medical University of Vienna detected microplastics in human feces across the globe. They revealed that each individual sample contained up to nine different types of plastic. To get an idea of how many plastic particles are in our gut, a research team, led by Kieran Cox at the University of Victoria, looked at the amount an average US citizen takes in from the air and food, each year. After evaluating twenty-six studies, they came up with an impressive number of 39,000 to 52,000 individual microplastic particles in the gastrointestinal tract. If we add the amount of nanoplastic particles we breathe in, we get a sum of around 74,000 to

121,000 particles per person per year. In reality, the number is probably much higher because only specific foods, such as sugar, salt, beer, honey, and seafood were studied. These foods accounted for only 15% of the average calorie intake. A person who drinks beverages from plastic bottles adds another 90,000 particles per year compared to someone who drinks tap water, which only adds 4000 particles. Kieran Cox believes his study underestimates the problem; he says: "A lot of the items we considered are the ones you're eating raw. We haven't gotten to the layers and layers of plastic packaging," and he adds, "I think it's probably the case that more plastic is being added than we realize".

There is growing evidence that the complex chemical composition of plastic poses a threat of physical and chemical toxicity to humans and other living beings. These plastic compounds are full of harmful chemical additives such as flame retardants, plasticizers and stabilizers that are incorporated during the manufacture process. Many plastic packages leach these chemicals into the food and beverages we consume. Leaching also occurs when we touch soft-grip products, as the chemicals are absorbed through the skin. Bisphenol A (commonly known as BPA) is a chemical that has been used in plastic production since the 1960s and is very harmful even in small doses. There are many other substances whose chemical compounds are largely unknown. They pose a potential danger to us. When microplastic and nanoplastic particles enter the gastrointestinal tract, they are incorporated into the microbiome and can cause a change in the makeup of the microbial population. Some of these plastic particles can be metabolized by bacteria or trigger the immune system, leading to inflammation and oxidative stress. If this condition is sustained, it can lead to tissue damage and cancer. There is also a microbial community in the lungs, albeit a much smaller one than in the gut. This microbiome can be altered when nanoplastics enter the lungs via house dust, particles from the abrasion of road surfaces, upholstery, carpets, electronics, and toys.

The madness doesn't stop there, as manufacturers deliberately add so-called micro-beads to their products to make them clean, rub, stir and feel better when used. These micro-beads are found in products such as adhesives, electronics, 3D printing materials, paints, cosmetics, and personal care products like toothpaste and shampoo. Have you ever thought that the harmless-looking glitter in craft and make-up could pose a threat to our planet? Yes, they too are microplastics.

Any type of plastic can potentially break down into nanoplastic particles during manufacturing and consumer use. For example, facial scrubs, anti-wrinkle creams and lipsticks contain micro-beads. Some of the particles from these products enter our bodies directly through the skin, and the remaining particles end up in the sink or on tissues, and from there to wastewater or landfill. This process also applies to textiles made from microfiber, such as nylon and polyester, as the particles from these garments enter the wastewater system during washing. Sewage systems cannot handle nanoplastic particles, because they are so small, and release them into the environment via waterways. Although some countries such as Sweden, the UK, and New Zealand have banned micro-beads to reduce their impact, there are still some niches for manufacturers. Canada, for example, allows nanoplastics in non-prescription drugs and in some natural health products.

Today's packaging is made of various plastics to improve its functional properties. This can be for optical, mechanical, catalytic, and antimicrobial reasons. They prolong the freshness and shelf-life of many products. Since it is no longer possible to free our planet from microplastics and nanoplastics, you can help to minimize additional plastic waste by choosing alternative products or avoiding plastics altogether. There are many ways to replace plastic products with more sustainable ones. By becoming aware of this problem, you can change your shopping habits.

There are already many fresh foods that are contaminated with plastic. I draw your attention to the popular, inconspicuous, and harmless-looking sea salt, because it is an excellent example of how we are still unaware of the full extent of the environmental pollution in our daily lives. We consume this salt in the belief that we are doing something good for our bodies. At the same time, we ignore the fact that it is often harvested in heavily contaminated areas. Researchers found that salt from the ocean and lagoons contains large amounts of microplastic and nanoplastic particles. According to a German study, there is no significant difference, in the concentration of these particles, between products from heavily polluted countries like China and Indonesia and the expensive French fleur de sel.

Another example of our ignorance concerns honey. Bees transport pollen and non-pollen-containing particles into their hives. During honey production, other microparticles can get into the product. Some producers package honey in plastic containers, with the result that honey may not be as beneficial as we would like to believe. Interestingly, a study on honey observed that unrefined honey has a much higher degree of contamination than processed and filtered honey. When choosing honey, it is no longer a question of whether it is contaminated or not, but to what extent. Considering the extent of gastrointestinal problems, one might wonder if Paracelsus, the famous medical scholar of the late Middle Ages, was not right when he said: "The dose makes the poison".

It always amazes me that many people do not make the connection between the polluted environment and our health problems. It's like deliberately putting poison in your food and pretending everything is fine. Fortunately, there is a growing awareness that agriculture must be environmentally conscious and sustainable. Soil regeneration, farmer welfare and chemical-free products for consumers are often part of this process. All over the world, there are projects large and small that you can support, whether directly or through your shopping habits. A visit to the farmer's market is a good start, but it's best to ask the market vendors where the produce comes from and how it was grown.

# IMMUNE SYSTEM

We cannot look at the digestive system in isolation, as there is an infinite interplay of processes that can influence it. A key player in this regard is the immune system. No part of the body is excluded from its surveillance. From the moment we are born, our bone marrow is the nursery for many specialized immune cells. After expert training, these cells are released to patrol the body. Without these hard-working soldiers, substances from the outside world would constantly enter the inner body unhindered. Their job is to screen for any potentially harmful pathogens such as bacteria, viruses, parasites, fungi, abnormal or cancerous cells, and eliminate them to maximize the body's survival.

The immune system has various strategies to protect the body. The first line of defense against non-self pathogens is the innate immune system. This system is present at birth. The skin, stomach acid, mucus and enzymes in the tears are its tools to build barriers against invaders. When invaders do manage to get into the body, this immune system recruits and activates all the cells needed to limit their spread. Its protective style is a bit rough. Everything that gets in its way, or looks a little strange, comes under attack. It is not uncommon for healthy tissue to be caught in the crossfire. If necessary, the innate immune system awakens the adaptive immune system to help on the ground.

The adaptive immune system is the second line of defense. Its tools are antibody receptors (immunoglobulins) with which it tries to protect the body. Its strategy is more sophisticated, as it usually distinguishes well between self and foreign bodies. Compared to the immediate and short-term response of the innate immune system, the adaptive immune response is long-lasting, highly specific and has a long-term memory. It can learn and remember that specific pathogens pose a danger to the body. The flip side of this is that it can make mistakes and attack healthy body cells. When this happens, inflammation and autoimmune diseases can develop.

Autoimmune diseases can be life-threatening and may last a lifetime. It is still not entirely clear why they occur. To some degree, everyone has autoimmune reactions, but they are not necessarily harmful. However, millions of people around the world are less fortunate, as they have one or more of the estimated hundred different autoimmune diseases. Well-known autoimmune diseases are type 1 diabetes, lupus, multiple sclerosis, ulcerative colitis, rheumatoid arthritis, and celiac disease. Sadly, many people suffer for years before receiving a correct diagnosis, as some autoimmune diseases are rare. Women are particularly suscep-tible to this type of disease; the reason could be related to their two main sex hormones, estrogen and progesterone. It is not uncommon for an autoimmune disease to run in the family, but it may take a different form for each member. For example, a mother has celiac disease, her sister has psoriasis, and her daughter has lupus.

The National Institute of Environmental Health Sciences believes that an autoimmune disease is an interaction between genetics and the environment. Influences include low birth weight and exposure to UV light, asbestos chemicals such as trichloroethylene - commonly used in cosmetics - and mercuric chloride, found in disinfectants and formerly used in solutions for analogue photography. Regular unprotected contact with these types of chemicals may be enough to trigger a liver-spe-cific autoimmune response. Cleaning products, paint thinners and nail polish are just a few of thousands of products that have contributed to systemic sclerosis – an autoimmune disease of the connective tissues. It seems that resistance to infection and susceptibility to autoimmune diseases are closely linked. An immune system that can respond more aggressively to infection is considered "strong" and could predispose a person to autoimmune disease.

Dr. Sarah Ballantyne, a medical biophysicist and creator of The Paleo Mom website, explains in one of her blogs that the immune system has a supportive relationship with the liver. When the liver is overloaded, it gets help from the immune system to process toxins. In return, the liver helps the immune system fight off unwanted guests. In both cases, inflammation may occur as these actions can contribute to overstimulation of the immune system. She adds that with a nutrient-poor diet and genetic predisposition, there is a higher risk of the immune system attacking healthy cells. Based on her research, she concludes that intestinal permeability (leaky gut) precedes the onset of this disease.

Testing for food intolerances can be a way to get more information about your condition, as it can reveal foods that trigger an immune response. Many of these tests use a technique called ELISA (enzyme-linked immunosorbent assay), which measures immunoglobulin, antibodies, antigens, and proteins. Some companies require a dried blood spot collection that can be done at home. It involves pricking your finger and drawing some blood on a piece of paper. This procedure is not quite child-friendly, as I experienced firsthand with my son. Other tests require a complete blood serum collection conducted by a nurse or a doctor.

A distinction is made between food intolerance responses that involve the digestive system and food allergy reactions that affect the immune system. The first situation occurs when the digestive system has difficulty breaking down certain foods. Perhaps it lacks a particular enzyme, is sensitive to food additives or has problems with the natural structure of the food itself. A true food allergy can be life-threatening because it causes the immune system to overreact. To defend against unwanted foods, the adaptive immune system activates antibodies and releases chemicals, sometimes triggering a hefty reaction. These antibodies, also known as immunoglobulins, are measured during an allergy and food intolerance test.

# IMMUNOGLOBULIN

There are five different classes of immunoglobulin:

* Immunoglobulin M (IgM) is the first on the scene to fight off infections. However, it provides only short-term protection and is soon replaced by IgG.

* Immunoglobulin G (IgG) is the most abundant type of antibody found in all body fluids, including blood. It is usually formed during an initial infection or other antigen exposure. It binds to viruses, bacteria, fungi and other microorganisms to protect the body. A deficiency of IgG, which may be caused by age, malnutrition, chemotherapy or long-term treatment with corticosteroids, can make you susceptible to leaky gut.

* Immunoglobulin A (IgA) is produced in large quantities every day, and is found primarily in the saliva, tears, respiration, and gastric secretions. It provides protection against infections in the mucosal membranes of the gastrointestinal tract and respiratory tract. Babies receive the first dose of IgA from their mothers during breastfeeding. Overly elevated IgG and IgA levels can be a sign of inflammatory bowel diseases.

* Immunoglobulin E (IgE) is associated with hypersensitivity or true allergies that can be triggered by cow's milk, peanuts, pollen, bees, latex, or other substances. The allergic reaction usually occurs within hours of exposure and can be severe or even fatal, (anaphylactic shock). There are more than 170 foods that can cause an allergy. Children are more susceptible than adults.

* Immunoglobulin D (IgD) is currently the least known antibody and is found in small amounts in the blood.

Your healthcare provider may test you for IgG food intolerance to get more information on your condition. These tests usually look at one to three hundred food items. Some companies offer special tests for Asian or vegetarian diets. For an additional fee, the lab can look for yeast and fungi, such as *Candida*, or markers for histamine intolerances. At first glance, it sounds like a good idea to identify foods that are causing you problems, but it can also create false expectations as the results are not as easy to interpret as you might think. There is a possibility that some highlighted foods do not really pose a problem for you, or conversely, foods that you know are problematic might not be highlighted. Gluten and dairy products are a good example. If you have not eaten these foods in a sufficient quantity every day for at least one month prior to the test, they may not show up as a concern. The American Academy of Allergy Asthma & Immunology says there is insufficient evidence that an IgG food intolerance test can diagnose food allergies or food intolerances. They advise against making serious changes to your diet based on these tests as the presence of IgG is a normal response of the immune system to food and may be a sign of its tolerance. Instead, they recommend consulting an allergist or immunologist for a proper diagnosis and treatment.

My doctor recommended that I take an IgG food intolerance test to broaden my food spectrum, since I reacted to most of the foods I ate. The result of the 300-item test revealed forty different problematic foods, of which about ten were particularly of concern. I eliminated all of these foods from my diet for a while. This approach helped me focus on the foods I could eat instead of eliminating more than I actually needed. This test was the first indication that I had a problem with gluten, which later turned out to be celiac disease. One rather unusual food item that was highlighted caused me a lot of trouble. A herbalist prepared a special tincture for my SIBO treatment. At first I was puzzled that this remedy made my symptoms worse. He changed the formula a few times, but nothing seemed to work until I checked my long list of food intolerances, and there was the culprit: nettle.

Sometimes it is helpful to avoid certain foods for a while, as this gives the body a break from substances it can't handle well. Please, don't reduce your diet to a mere handful of ingredients. One study shows that people with inflammatory bowel disease, such as Crohn's disease and ulcerative colitis, often suffer from nutritional deficiencies because they have overly restricted the variety of their diet in the hope of relieving their symptoms. If you are having difficulty creating or maintaining a balanced diet, you can consult a nutritionist.

Even when it comes to food allergies, the traditional avoidance diet has been reconsidered in recent years. The general trend is towards a varied diet to nourish the microbiome, which is especially important for the young, as it helps to build immune intolerance. Of course, any omission or addition of foods must be considered individually and cannot be recommended across the board.

---

Believe me, I've been in the situation where I only had a handful of foods to choose from. It was a very stressful and lonely place. When I started my health journey, I reduced my diet to three foods and added a new one every four days. If a reaction occurred, such as bloating, constipation, skin issues, I would drop the new food. I used this method for six months, and by then I had about fifteen foods on hand that I thought were safe. For a while, I felt great. But very slowly, and almost unnoticed, the old bloated me crept back. How could this be? What went wrong? I was devastated and my mental state was not good at that time. Looking back, I wouldn't do this kind of diet again because, knowing what I know today, it probably did me more harm than good as I wasn't eating enough variety of food to promote a healthy diversity in my microbiome. On top of that, I also ate a lot of different kinds of meat, but I didn't know that I had developed a mammalian meat allergy (red meats), from a tick. If you have been bitten by a tick, you should consider a blood test for alpha-gal, short for galactose-1,3-galactose. It triggers the immune system and can also cause anaphylactic reactions, which can be life-threatening. If you test positive, you must avoid foods that come from mammals, such as dairy products or gelatins (supplements and confectionery). Wine can also pose a risk, as it is often clarified with dairy products.

# LEAKY GUT

Science is just beginning to unravel the extent to which the microbiome and the immune system influence each other. So far, we know that the relationship between these two important systems has an enormous impact on our health and the body's homeostasis – the biological system and its self-regulating processes that aim to keep the body in a stable state to ensure survival.

An unsolved mystery is how the immune system can distinguish between resident gut microbes and pathogens. It is still puzzling how single or groups of bacterial species can affect the host. Apparently, researchers have recognized that a damaged and impaired gastrointestinal tract, including the various levels of the mucosa and epithelial cells, contributes to immune system dysfunction. These epithelial cells are a densely packed, fine row of cells located at the interface between the inner and outer worlds of the body. This lightweight protective shield, with filtration, absorption, and secretion functions, acts as a receptor that collects and transmits information to the brain. Epithelial cells must distinguish between harmful and beneficial substances and organisms. Anything that passes through their barrier can enter the blood stream.

These epithelial cells have nothing to hold on to except a fibrous matrix called the basement membrane, which is made of collagen, enzymes, and proteins. This provides a structure for the tight epithelial cell bond. When a bond weakens, a gap is created and food molecules, toxins and pathogens can enter the blood stream, directly into the arms of the immune system. If this process occurs in the intestine, it is commonly known as increased intestinal permeability or leaky gut. Other names associated with this condition are "metabolic endotoxemia" and "hyperpermeability".

You may wonder how it can happen that the intestines leak, and toxins enter the bloodstream, causing autoimmune diseases, and other diseases such as Alzheimer's and cancer. Scientists believe that the diversity of the microbiome had to be affected first. A low-fiber diet, high in sugar and fat contributes to an increase in permeability. This type of diet eliminates health-promoting microbial strains and allows more harmful strains to flourish, blocking the absorption of nutrients. Epithelial cells depend on the supply of energy through nutrients to maintain their health.

Kiran Krishnan, a research microbiologist, and co-founder of Nu Science Trading and Microbiome Labs, explains that the next step in the development of leaky gut is when microbes begin to eat away the inner protective barrier of the mucosa, leading to erosion of some sections. In these pockets microbes make a safe home for themselves and invite all kinds of guests to join their little enclave. Once they have eaten through the mucosa, they reach the epithelial cells and damage or destroy them, triggering immune responses. Mr. Krishnan says this process is responsible for many food sensitivities and is a major cause of chronic health issues.

To a certain extent, it is quite normal for the intestines to have some permeability – this should not be a cause for concern. Some people are more susceptible than others to the development of leaky gut due to a genetic predisposition or a sensitive digestive system. Other causes include alcohol consumption, pathogens such as *E. coli*, or the regular use of NSAIDs. There are many diseases associated with this condition, including autoimmune diseases such as celiac disease, chronic inflammatory bowel disease, Crohn's disease, arthritis, type 1 diabetes, multiple sclerosis, lupus, and dermatological conditions such as eczema, psoriasis and acne.

There are several functional tests to detect leaky gut. First, the sugar absorption tests of lactulose and mannitol. Each of these sugar molecules allows assessment of different areas of gut health. Lactulose absorption indicates gut damage, while mannitol absorption is used to measure small intestine function. These tests can be ordered through your healthcare provider and performed at home. After drinking a prepared solution, urine is collected in a bag over a six-hour period. A small sample of the collected fluid is sent to the laboratory. If the result shows an increase in lactulose in the urine, it means that this larger sugar molecule was able to pass through the epithelial cells, indicating intestinal permeability. The mannitol test has an additional advantage in that it can detect malabsorption.

Zonulin is a protein that controls the connection between individual epithelial cells. When the body produces too much of this protein, the openings between the cells can enlarge, allowing unwanted particles to pass through. A common trigger for an increase in zonulin is gluten, particularly its gliadin protein (a prominent protein of wheat), and an excess of bacteria in the small intestine. Researchers found that zonulin is elevated in a variety of diseases such as autoimmune, neurodegenerative and metabolic diseases. To determine if you have a problem with this protein, you can undergo a blood test to check your zonulin levels. This test is often used to monitor whether a gluten-free diet is sufficient for a celiac disease patient. Chris Kresser, the co-director of the California Center for Functional Medicine and creator of chriskresser.com, doubts the reliability of this method and suggests examining the cause of leaky gut rather than the symptoms. It is open to debate whether it makes sense to spend money on a leaky gut test if you already have several health problems such as SIBO, IBS, food sensitivity, nutrient deficiency, chronic stress, intestinal infections, or an immune system disorder, because all these disorders are an indicator of leaky gut. If testing is required, Chris Kresser prefers the lactulose and mannitol sugar test or an Array 2 test instead of the zonulin test. The Array 2 is an intestinal permeability antigenic sensor test. This technology can detect barrier damage before dysfunction occurs. It identifies antibodies (occludin and zonulin) and the immune response to lipopolysaccharides (LPS), large molecules located in the membrane of certain bacteria. Compared to the lactulose and mannitol sugar test, it is designed to measure nutrient absorption rather than intestinal permeability. There are other interesting Array tests available, such as Array 3 for wheat and gluten sensitivity, or Array 4 for testing cross-reactive foods.

After the irritating foods have been eliminated from the diet, it is usually time to focus on restoring the intestinal mucosa. For this reason, dietary supplements and therapeutic diets are an integral part of an individual health plan created by your healthcare provider. This often includes digestive enzymes, probiotics, and L-glutamine, an amino acid that is naturally produced by the body. For various reasons, such as a genetic predisposition, some people are unable to produce enough glutamine. Glutamine plays an important role in many bodily functions such as tissue production, intestinal barrier, inflammation regulation, stress responses, and for the immune system. It is not surprising that the gastrointestinal system is one of the main consumers of this valuable amino acid, and within this system the small intestine requires particularly high amounts. There is controversy within the scientific community as to whether glutamine supplementation is beneficial in intestinal diseases. In clinical trials, a positive result has been noted during the flare-up phase of inflammatory bowel disease with glutamine administration. A recent double-blind, placebo-controlled study on IBS patients concluded that eight weeks of oral glutamine therapy effectively reduced symptoms, especially in IBS-D patients who also suffered from intestinal permeability. On the other hand, some scientists question the necessity of taking glutamine supplements, as it is not always clear whether a person has a deficiency or not. I would like to emphasize that everyone may respond differently to treatments. For some people glutamine supplementation works wonders; for others, it doesn't do anything. Although it is sometimes tempting, I do not recommend self-treatment with this amino acid because the gastrointestinal tract is so complex. Consult a specialist for SIBO and IBS, even if it means having to grasp the nettle and pay a lot of money.

# NATURAL CHEMICALS

Some plant food can make life difficult for people as they cause aller-gy-like symptoms such as skin rashes, stuffy nose, hay fever, and asthma when consumed. Other symptoms can include stomach and intestinal problems, immune system and hormone dysfunctions. The reason for all these issues can be the presence of naturally occurring chemicals such as salicylates, oxalates, tannins, histamines, and lectins in these foods. I would like to introduce you to three of these natural chemicals.

## HISTAMINE

Histamine is produced by the immune system to protect the body from pathogens. It also regulates gastric acid secretion and acts as a neurotransmitter, sending messages between cells. When the immune system detects a threat, it sends signals to mast cells in the skin, lungs, nose, mouth, intestines, and blood to release stored histamine. Histamine is like the bouncer of a nightclub who is responsible for opening the door to individual guests. In our bodies, it encourages permeability for various reasons, for example, to allow white blood cells and some proteins to enter and get the party started. It also promotes blood flow and uses its repertoire of functions to ward off perceived danger by causing pseudo-allergic reactions such as diarrhea, headache, congestion, runny nose, sneezing, itchy or watery eyes, asthma, low blood pressure, irregular heart rate, hives, rashes, swelling, bloating, flushing. Sometimes the owner of the nightclub, the immune system, is a bit overcautious and hires too many bouncers, mistakenly assuming that the harmless crowd is getting out of control. It's like the bouncers are having a punk slam-dance party and causing far more trouble, leading to an increase of inflammation. More protectors are needed – until things get completely out of hand. This whole situation can lead to histamine sensitivity or intolerance.

A healthy person can efficiently detoxify histamine through the intestinal enzyme diamine oxidase (DAO). However, some people do not have enough of this histamine-degrading enzyme, or they accumulate histamine in the body for other reasons such as genetic susceptibility or a compromised gut. Middle-aged people and, in particular, women in the premenstrual phase are more susceptible to this problem. In conditions such as dysbiosis, IBS, SIBO and SIFO, histamine accumulates because bacteria and yeasts produce this chemical as a by-product. Histamine intolerance differs from other food intolerance in that it is caused by the accumulation of histamine rather than the release of it. Symptoms may appear immediately after a meal or up to a day or two later.

As you may have painfully experienced, many plants and insect venoms contain histamine, which can cause swelling, itching or pain on contact. An antihistamine is usually given to provide relief.

Conventional foods and beverages also contain histamine. The amount varies greatly depending on storage and maturation of the food. Particularly high levels of histamine are in fermented foods such as sauerkraut and fish sauce, but it is also found in most cheeses, yeast products, nightshade vegetables (such as eggplant and tomatoes), spinach, coffee, chocolate, marinated fish, cured and canned meats, vinegar, tomato sauce/ketchup, and alcoholic beverages such as red wine. All these foods should be avoided if you have a problem with histamine. In fact, all convenience and semi-prepared foods should be consumed with caution because bacteria can get into them during manufacture, releasing histamine long before the food is considered unsafe. Freshly prepared meals that are eaten on the spot are the safest.

Some foods, even if they are low in histamine, can stimulate the release of histamine in the body. These foods are the so-called histamine liberators. Depending on your sensitivity, you may want to avoid bananas, citrus fruit such as lemon, lime, and grapefruit, egg whites, legumes like lentils and chickpeas, licorice, pork, shellfish and various nuts and seeds such as cashews, peanuts, walnuts, and sunflower seeds.

Some medications can also interact with histamine or block the DAO enzyme. It is worth reviewing them and discussing any further steps with your healthcare provider.

Histamine intolerance is often misinterpreted or underestimated. Sometimes people are considered hypochondriacs because their symptoms cannot be clearly attributed because DAO or histamine levels do not necessarily correlate with their symptoms. Whether histamine is a problem cannot be determined with an IgE allergy test. Currently, the only way to find out if this chemical is causing symptoms is to follow a strict, low-histamine diet for an extended period of time. Since almost all foods contain some amount of histamine, the focus is on eliminating foods high in histamine from the diet. To reduce histamine formation, cooked and leftover food should be placed in the refrigerator or frozen as soon as possible. It is challenging to combine a low-histamine diet with an already restricted SIBO or IBS diet – possibly gluten-free diet as well. If you find yourself in this situation, check out Dr. Jacobi's Bi-Phasic Diet for SIBO and histamine intolerance and/or consult a qualified nutritionist to ensure that you are consuming adequate nutrients. At a later point in your health journey, you can try to reintroduce histamine rich foods to your diet, as tolerance to histamine seems to improve significantly after gastrointestinal recovery.

## OXALATES

Like all living beings, plants have a metabolism. Oxalic acid and its relatives, the oxalates, play a major role in this. It is not entirely understood how, but these natural chemicals are essential for specific functions within plants. They regulate calcium and iron levels, act as plant protection agents, support tissues, and detoxify heavy metals. An excess of oxalic acid can be toxic to humans because we lack an enzyme that breaks it down. When oxalate enters the body, it is normally excreted before it can cause us harm. It should be noted that as it passes through the body, it binds with minerals such as calcium, magnesium, potassium and sodium, possibly leading to nutrient deficiencies. This may explain why people with malabsorption are more susceptible to oxalate toxicity, which is also associated with inflammation, joint pain, and leaky gut. When oxalate binds with calcium, it forms insoluble calcium oxalate, which can cause kidney stones and crystals. To make things worse, yeasts and bacteria such as *Candida* and *Aspergillus* species increase oxalate levels.

In our modern life, oxalate is found in cleaning products, bleach, and baking powder. Contact or ingestion in concentrated form can cause severe burns, nausea, severe gastroenteritis, or even kidney failure. Special attention should be paid to plants that contain large amounts of oxalates such as buckwheat, amaranth, taro, yam, sweet potato, beetroot, sorrel, spinach, rhubarb, radishes, berries, sesame seeds, nuts (especially almonds and pecans), turmeric, grains, and legumes. The distribution of oxalates within the plant is uneven, with the substance being highest in the leaves, moderate in seeds, and lowest in the stems. The concentration also depends on where and when it was grown, and its maturity. Maybe your mother warned you as a child not to chew on rhubarb leaves or eat uncooked beans. Now you know the reason: they contain large amounts of oxalates.

Not every dietary fad is necessarily healthy; that includes green smoothies, big raw salads, and Buddha bowls. These foods are full of oxalates as they contain mostly raw ingredients, such as kale, chard, spinach, berries, or almonds. Preparing foods in a certain way helps to reduce oxalates, particularly when it comes to pulses and beans. Soaking overnight and cooking thoroughly until soft seems to do the trick. The disadvantage of this method is that it destroys many nutrients. The sprouting technique is different because it preserves nutrients while reducing oxalates. It can be applied to legumes, seeds, nuts, and grains; but beware, kidney beans should not be sprouted and consumed, because they are poisonous when eaten raw. A healthy person should not avoid oxalate-containing foods, as most of them provide a variety of nutrients. The earlier-mentioned organic acids test (OAT) can detect the presence of oxalates. If you have to follow a low oxalate diet, it is advisable not to eliminate all oxalate-containing foods at once. Start slowly, otherwise symptoms may get worse. A dietary supplement such as calcium citrate can support the treatment as it absorbs oxalates.

## SALICYLATES

Much like oxalate, salicylate acts as protection against insect attacks and plant diseases. The WHO included salicylate as one of the most effective and safest medicines on its Model List of Essential Medicines. It is used to treat warts, psoriasis, dandruff, acne, and ringworm. An interesting property is that it can help remove the outer layer of skin cells. Many health, beauty, and cosmetic products contain a natural or synthetic form of salicylate. A well-known and widely used salicylic medication is aspirin (acetylsalicylic acid). It has an analgesic and antipyretic effect, but is also one of the most common causes of salicylate overdose.

In some people, a diet containing salicylate may mimic aspirin toxicity. This can happen out of the blue. Dr. Donna Beck, a well-known naturopath who is sensitive to salicylate herself, points out that salicylates are more likely to cause problems when the immune system is weakened, during bacterial overgrowth (hello SIBO and IBS!), injuries, or hormonal changes due to menopause. Normally, the body neutralizes high levels of salicylate with carbon dioxide, but if it cannot do this, the salicylate can cause changes in the respiratory system. In the worst-case scenario, it can trigger hyperventilation. This strong physical reaction is provoked to restore balance in the body. Dr. Beck explains that salicylate itself can form acids, which in turn create more salicylates. In addition, acid-forming bacteria can contribute to an increase in salicylates. In this vicious circle, the body quickly consumes minerals such as calcium, magnesium, and potassium as it struggles to cope with this acid load.

People with leaky gut or impaired liver enzymes may be more susceptible to salicylate intolerance because they cannot metabolize this chemical properly. Symptoms of intolerance include ringing in the ears, drop in blood pressure, nausea, hyperventilation, vertigo, headaches, abdominal pain, intestinal inflammation, colitis, diarrhea, and swelling of hands, feet, and face. In many cases, the skin is affected with a change of color, itching, irritation, rash, or hives. Some people develop a sun sensitivity or respiratory issues such as nasal congestion, polyposis, rhinitis, asthma, or breathing difficulties. A severe salicylate poisoning can lead to anaphylaxis. To counteract an excess of salicylate in the body, especially in the case of poisoning, Dr. Beck recommends drinking sodium bicarbonate mixed with water.

In nature, salicylates occur in higher concentrations in unripe fruit and vegetables. Unfortunately, it is common practice in the food industry that fruit and vegetables are harvested far too early, which puts us as consumers in a dilemma. Other foods that are high in salicylate include olive oil, coconut oil, pineapples, dates, guava, cloves, honey, peanuts, zucchini, radish, eggplant, broad beans, chicory, herbs and spices like turmeric, cayenne, ginger, curry, Chinese five spices.

A product called Wintergreen oil, also known as Boxberry, Canada Tea, Mountain Tea, and Gaultheria, should be taken with caution. It is often used for digestive problems such as bloating, and to increase gastric juices, and also for headaches, nerve pain, arthritis, ovarian pain, and menstrual cramps. Be extremely careful with it because as little as one ounce (30 ml) of this oil is equivalent to about 170 aspirin tablets for adults and can lead to poisoning.

Currently, the only way to know if you are salicylate intolerant is to reduce the intake by avoiding salicylate-containing foods and medications. Once the physically stored salicylate is eliminated, the body can be provoked again, preferably under medical supervision, to determine if and when intolerance occurs. An epicutaneous test can determine if a reaction to salicylate-containing sunscreens and other cosmetics could be the cause of any skin problems.

If you have a salicylate intolerance, it is important to follow a low salicylate diet for a while. Using bone broth (histamine!) and mushrooms helps to break down this chemical in the body. Actually, any high-sulfur foods may help. Herbs such as fennel and marshmallow root are excellent to support the kidneys. If you are in the first treatment phase of SIBO, or have not started a treatment yet, marshmallow root may not be a good choice for you as it can promote overgrowth of bacteria in the small intestine, according to Dr. Jacobi. With salicylate intolerance, it is advisable to avoid acidic foods such as salt. For this reason, it may also be wise to check the pH of the water at home to make sure it is not too alkaline or too acidic. Fortunately, Dr. Beck gives hope to people suffering from this intolerance. In an interview with Dr. Jacobi, she mentions that it is possible to overcome and reverse this condition. Once your metabolism has returned to normal, you can slowly reintroduce foods. It's worth asking the question: Why did your metabolism go off the rails in the first place?

Sue Dengate, a psychology graduate and former teacher, discovered firsthand that salicylates, amines and food chemicals were greatly affecting her children's behavior. Working with the Royal Prince Alfred Hospital in Australia, she developed a diet called FAILSAFE, which stands for "Free of Additives, Low in Salicylates, Amines and Flavor Enhancer". It was originally developed to treat attention deficit hyperactivity disorder (ADHD) in children, but is by no means limited to this condition. Her first book *Different Kids. Growing Up with Attention Deficit Disorder* was followed by *Fed Up: Understanding How Food Affects Your Child and What You Can Do About It* and *The Failsafe Cookbook: Reducing Food Chemicals for Calm, Happy Families.* Together with her scientist husband Dr. Howard Dengate, she created the Food Intolerance Network that can be found on their Fed Up website.

# CONCEPT SUMMARY

» Inflammation is a physical signal indicating that something in the body needs attention. There are many different reasons for the development of inflammatory processes, which include microbial infections. More difficult to recognize are low-grade inflammations that can lead to chronic inflammation and are often associated with autoimmune diseases.

» The pollution of our planet by plastic products not only affects our environment, but also humans. There are thousands of different substances in plastic - a chemical time bomb - which makes it difficult to predict interactions. Scientists know that plastic substances are already altering the microbiome, putting health at risk.

» Leaky gut is a condition that indicates damage to the intestinal mucosa and epithelial cells, which are the physical barrier between the inside and outside of the body. Once this condition occurs, passers-by such as microbes and proteins can freely enter the bloodstream and cause immune system reactions.

» The immune system is a whole-body surveillance system that tries to fight off invaders such as bacteria and viruses. Sometimes it mistakenly attacks the body's cells and stores the memory of this action for the future. To clear this memory and activate the body's self-healing process, it is important to avoid all foods that could trigger the immune system.

» Endogenous chemicals such as histamines, oxalates, and salicylates can become out of balance due to gastrointestinal disorders and hormonal changes, leading to food intolerances, irritation of the intestinal mucosa, respiratory issues, and even poisoning.

# DIETARY CONSIDERATIONS

In the past, for me, eating wasn't about satisfying my hunger, but rather about taste experiences and favorite foods. My ignorance has not necessarily helped my body stay in good health. After I was diagnosed with IBS and SIBO, I had to do a major rethink. It took me a while to figure out the best way to nourish myself, because there wasn't enough information available at the time. To give you a better start, I'll take you on a nutritional journey for a better understanding of what to watch out for, followed by a description of common diets for SIBO and IBS. In my experience, following a strict short-term diet and searching for recipes on the Internet or in cookbooks is not enough for a sustainable dietary change. It is better to know the basics of nutrition and apply these guidelines every day. To begin, let's look at the three most important macronutrients needed to sustain life: Carbohydrates, proteins, and fats.

## CARBOHYDRATES, PROTEINS, AND FATS

Carbohydrates are probably the most abundant and widespread organic matter on earth. They come almost exclusively from plants but are also found in milk and, in small amounts, in red meat. The consumption of carbohydrates enables the body to utilize glucose. It is the body's main source of energy and is especially important for the brain. Any excess of glucose is stored in the liver and muscles but can also convert into body fat. When we eat carbohydrates sugar levels rise, and the pancreas secretes a hormone called insulin. This hormone helps to transport sugar molecules to the rest of the body for energy production and storage. If this process occurs too quickly, we will soon feel hungry again. If this process is slowed down it provides a more sustainable energy.

Carbohydrates are classified into simple and complex sugars. The simple sugar molecule is usually sweeter than the complex version. You may have heard the term FODMAP. This is an abbreviation for

Fermentable sugars: **O**ligosaccharides, **D**isaccharides, **M**onosaccharides **A**nd **P**olyols. They gained popularity thanks to the low-FODMAP diet developed by Australia's Monash University. In this diet, foods are divided into groups according to their respective sugar molecule. The approach is to eliminate each group for a period of time to determine which one is causing symptoms. This diet is widely used for IBS but is also helpful for SIBO. You'll find more information about this diet in the chapter "diets".

Sugar molecules are a bit like LEGO bricks. Using the analogy to these single, double, and multiple building blocks, they are defined according to their number of atoms and their structure. A sugar that consists of only one molecule is called monosaccharide ("mono" means one) and is also known as "simple" sugar. It does not need to be digested as it can be absorbed directly into the bloodstream and spike our sugar levels. There are three common types of these simple sugar "building blocks": glucose, galactose and fructose. Glucose is also known as dextrose and occurs naturally in fruits and vegetables. Galactose is found in milk, while fructose is found in fruit and honey and used as a sweetener in processed foods. When two of the simple sugar molecules are combined, they form disaccharides. They are like a "double brick" that comes in different varieties.

The three most common disaccharides are sucrose, lactose, and maltose. Sucrose is found in household sugar derived from sugar cane, and in vegetables like beet. People with sucrose intolerance lack the enzyme sucrase-isomaltose. Not only do they have problems digesting sucrose but may also have problems with starch as found in potatoes. Lactose is an essential component of dairy products. Earlier in human evolution, milk was digestible only by infants, but humans have developed an enzyme that allows them to consume it into adulthood. Since the adaptation of this enzyme is still quite young in the evolution of modern humans, many people today have problems tolerating dairy products. The third disaccharide sugar is maltose, which is found in cereals, beer, and confectionery. It is often used as a sweetener in chocolate to balance the bitterness of the cocoa bean. Plants produce maltose naturally when the plant's starch is broken down for seed growth.

As with real LEGO, where you can assemble the building blocks endlessly and let your imagination run wild, monosaccharides and disaccharides can be combined in myriad ways. Chains from three to several hundred sugar molecules make a complex sugar. These complex structures must be digested and do not cause blood sugar levels to rise as quickly. Oligos are small chains of monosaccharides. Most of them are rich in fiber and poorly absorbed in the small intestine. This feature benefits the bacteria in the large intestine, which is why oligos are considered prebiotics. In many people, oligos are the culprit of IBS symptoms such as bloating, abdominal discomfort, and impaired motility. In a healthy person, oligos are usually not a problem as they might only cause a little wind. Two of these oligos are fructans and galacto-oligos (GOS). Fructans are widely found in fruit, grains, pulses, nuts, and vegetables. GOS, on the other hand, is mainly found in legumes such as chickpeas, lentils, and beans. Human breast milk contains more than two hundred different oligos and is essential for healthy brain development in infants. It not only ensures a pleasantly soft bowel movement, but also protects the child from disease.

The last of the FODMAPs is polyols, sugar alcohols. Polyols are naturally present in many fruits and vegetables, including stone fruits, mushrooms, and avocados. The food industry adds them to chewing gum, mints, and diabetic products because they taste less sweet. The most common polyols are maltitol, xylitol, sorbitol, and mannitol – of which the latter two often trigger IBS symptoms. Like fructose, polyols can also stress the intestine by drawing in water (osmotic effect) and causing gas. Both conditions can make you look like you are pregnant. The severity of this condition may depend on how sensitive a person is and the number of polyols they have consumed.

For some people the fermentation of FODMAPs can lead to neurological symptoms such as confusion, slurred speech, memory loss and feeling "drunk". The solution to this problem is to eliminate the FODMAPs you are sensitive to and include more healthy fats in your diet.

> Monash University's Low FODMAP diet app is a fantastic tool that helped me become aware of these food groups. At first, using the app was like riding a bike with training wheels, but after a while I was able to get away from it and felt comfortable making my own food choices. I admit that not all of them were ideal – I guess that's part of the learning curve. Since this app is updated regularly, it's still a tool I turn to sometimes.

## PROTEIN

When you ask someone why we should consume protein, the answer is often "for creating more muscles". It is too simplistic to reduce this vital nutrient to that of developing biceps, as it maintains virtually every part and tissue of the body. When the protein we eat is digested, it is broken down into chemical "building blocks" called amino acids. These molecules consist of nitrogen, carbon, hydrogen and oxygen and enter the blood. Amino acids govern all cells by maintaining, building, and replacing them. They are also involved in enzyme and hormone production. Without amino acids nothing works, which is why they are so important for all living things.

Since amino acids cannot be stored in the body, they must be supplied daily through our diet. There are twenty in all, and nine of them are defined as essential. The other eleven have the misleading name "non-essential". Although we need them as well, an adult body can synthesize them. We are at risk of failing health if our bodies do not receive an adequate supply of all of them. A deficiency can affect all organs, the immune system and the gastrointestinal tract. Symptoms of inadequate amino acid intake include muscle and joint pain, insomnia, fatigue, moodiness, stress, altered skin and hair texture, and a constant craving for carbohydrates.

You may wonder how much protein you need. The quantity depends largely on individual factors such as age, gender, genes, body weight and stage of life. Generally, women should consume 46 grams and men 56 grams of protein per day. Pregnant women and adults who want to build more muscle, need a slightly higher amount. The same applies to children because their growth requires more. It is recommended to consume small amounts of high-quality protein over two or three meals a day to ensure an optimal supply of essential amino acids, nitrogen, and the building materials for the non-essential amino acids. To determine your personal needs, you can access the United States Department of Agriculture (USDA) calculator, which will give you a rough idea of whether your consumption is within the healthy range. As an alternative, you may like to consult a nutritionist who can give you a more comprehensive picture of your requirements. Sometimes we have a higher need for protein, for example during infections, fever, gastro-enteritis, after severe injuries, especially burns, or postoperative stress.

Although protein deficiency is rare in countries such as Australia, people with special food requirements, such as vegetarians and vegans, need to pay special attention to their intake. The same cautions apply to older people, as they are more susceptible to protein malnutrition. They often experience a lack of energy and appetite, leading consequently to weight loss. Scientists call it the "anorexia of aging". The cause may lie in numerous biological and physiological changes, such as hormonal imbalance, impaired body fluids, decrease in senses of smell and taste, chronic disorders, and mental illness. Besides alcoholism or an inadequate protein consumption - which may be due to a very restrictive diet - many diseases can cause a protein deficiency. These diseases promote the inability to digest and absorb dietary proteins. This is especially true of most chronic gastrointestinal disorders, such as inflammatory bowel diseases, IBS, and SIBO. In the latter cases, bacteria prevent adequate supply of protein or consume it themselves.

Animal-based foods are close to the biochemical structure of humans and provide all nine essential amino acids. This is not to say that plant sources are any less valuable. There are many excellent plant proteins from vegetables, nuts, whole grains, legumes, lentils, and soy. If you want to consume soy products choose the less processed products such as edamame, soybeans, traditionally made tofu and tempeh. Since most vegetable proteins are incomplete, which means that they lack one or more essential amino acid, it is advisable to eat different varieties every day to get enough. The idea that plant foods can only provide complete amino acids if they are combined in a certain way at each meal, such as legumes with rice, is outdated. It is okay if you eat a balanced diet every day.

Dr. Alan Desmond, a gastroenterologist from the Devon Gut Clinic, says a plant-based diet is rich in antioxidants and anti-inflammatories. It provides the body with a greater diversity of nutrition, fiber and a more stable microbiome than an omnivorous diet. Vegetarian and vegan diets promote improved carbohydrate metabolism, which in turn regulates glucose and energy homeostasis and supports gut epithelial barrier health. Although legumes, grains and seeds, including rice, are celebrated for their protein and fiber they can become a problem for some people. The reason is often the prolamin in these foods. Prolamin is a storage container for the protein in the seed. Soaking these foods overnight then preparing them as usual can ease this issue.

Long-term high-protein consumption may be counterproductive, or simply harmful. This is especially true for those with a meat-heavy diet without a wide variety of plant foods, as it promotes a pro-inflammatory environment. Also, high consumption of red meat increases the intake of saturated fats, which can lead to a higher risk of cardiovascular disease. Eating ham increases blood pressure and the risk of stroke due to its sodium content. It can even lead to calcium loss and subsequently osteoporosis. If you don't want to give up a meat-heavy diet, try to avoid processed meats that have been cured, salted, fermented, or smoked.

By 2050, the world's population could reach ten billion people, all of whom will need to be fed from this planet. We can no longer ignore the devastating impact of our eating habits on the environment. With each meal, our decisions have a positive or negative impact. Switching to a sustainable diet not only benefits our environment, but also our health. The World Recourse Institute recommends significantly reducing the consumption of beef, sheep and goat meat and moderate consumption of chicken, pork and farmed fish. With this in mind, switching to a mainly plant-based diet can be an excellent choice. Still, the 2019 Food, Planet, Health report from the EAT-Lancet Commission points out that it's not just meat that's taking a toll on the environment, but also eating too many root vegetables. In their recommendation, they point out that half of the plate should be vegetables or fruits. The other half should consist of whole grains, plant-based protein and unsaturated fats or oils. Optionally, a modest amount of animal protein is also acceptable.

Broths and stocks make a nutritious source of amino acids and minerals that can be incorporated into your diet. Across cultures, both foods are traditionally used as a remedy to strengthen the body when sick or weak. They can be made from chicken, fish, meat, and bones, as well as from mushrooms or vegetables, such as Bieler's broth, which is made from zucchini, French beans, celery, and parsley. Broth and stock are food relatives but not twins. A stock is always made from bones that have simmered for a long time. This process makes it rich in gelatin. A broth is made from meat or vegetables and is usually not strained before serving. When strained, it is usually used as a base for soups or sauces. Another variation is consommé, which is a perfectly clarified and concentrated form of stock or broth. All these foods are not a substitute for a full meal, but they can enrich your diet. Keep in mind, consuming broth and stock can cause bothersome symptoms in people who suffer from histamine intolerance. If you want to try them and don't know if you are among those affected, you should start gently to incorporate them into your diet.

For a comprehensive list of protein foods and their nutritional values, visit the USDA website. Beware that some protein-containing foods can cause allergic reactions or intolerances, which is especially true for milk, eggs, peanuts, soybeans, shellfish and tree nuts. Some people may find it difficult to incorporate enough protein into their diet. To counteract this problem a protein powder may be the solution. These powders are usually made from whey (be careful, it contains lactose!), peas or even crickets. They are mixed into drinks such as smoothies, sprinkled on cereal, or used in baking. There are no limits to your imagination. Make sure you buy an allergy-free product, meaning that it does not contain fillers like gluten, soy, nuts, eggs, and dairy. Opt for an organic product that has a "complete" protein with all amino acids.

If you suspect you may have a protein deficiency, ask your doctor for a "total protein" blood test. It measures the amount and concentration of two specific proteins: albumin and globulin. Albumin is produced in the liver and is responsible for preventing fluid leaking from the blood vessels. It also transports small molecules, hormones, vitamins, and drugs throughout the body. Albumin deficiency is associated with white lines on the nails (Muehrcke's lines) and liver disease. Globulins are a family of more than 500 proteins, including enzymes and antibodies, which are produced in the liver and, to some extent, in the immune system. The globulin level may indicate an inflammatory disorder or infection in the body.

Other options include testing for protein C and protein S. These tests measure how much clotting occurs in the blood. The blood's ability to clot is crucial because it prevents the body from bleeding too much after an injury. In the absence of these two proteins, clotting can occur even without injury, which can be life-threatening. The development of protein C depends on vitamin K. Deficiency of this vitamin is often found in alcoholic liver disease. In contrast, a lack of the protein S can cause deep vein thrombosis (DVT) in the arms or legs. There are certain situations in which there is a high risk of DVT including pregnancy, surgery, older age, or being very inactive, as in the case of long-distance flights. There is no cure for protein S deficiency other than taking blood thinning medications and/or making lifestyle changes to reduce the risk of clotting.

## FATS AND OILS

Evolution has led humans to prefer foods with fatty and sweet flavors because they provide a valuable source of energy. Fat takes longer to break down but is the most efficient form of energy. Each gram of fat provides about 9 calories, more than twice as much as protein and carbohydrates. It supports cell function, keeps us warm, and protects organs. It helps the body to absorb the fat soluble vitamins such as vitamin A, vitamin D, and vitamin E. The body also uses fat to synthesize hormones. Since fat is so important for the body, excess amounts are stored for later use under the skin and in the abdominal area - sometimes even in blood vessels or in organs.

Fat (lipid) metabolism is a sophisticated process that reminds me of a logistical system in which things are distributed, sorted, packed, unpacked, stored, and delivered. It works mainly in the stomach and in the upper part of the small intestine before its components can be converted into energy. When you eat a meal, say a burger, it is broken down and sorted into units. Special workers, the lipase digestive enzymes, take care of the pile of fat by breaking it down with the help of bile salts into smaller units. The goal is to break down fat into fatty acids. Fatty acids are the "building blocks" of fat. They are usually grouped together and classified according to their length into long-chain fatty acids (LCFAs), medium-chain fatty acids (MCFAs) and SCFAs.

Large amounts of fatty acids must be transported as triglycerides to avoid toxicity in the body. These units not only contain fatty acids but also cholesterol molecules, phospholipids, and proteins. These newly formed packages - called chylomicrons - are ready to cross the aqueous environment of the lymphatic system to enter the blood. Their destination is the cell where they unpack all their triglyceride goodies and deliver them to the cells to nourish tissues and muscles. After completing their mission, the chylomicrons begin to shrink and become lipoprotein. There are several classes of circulating lipoproteins, each of which has its own characteristic protein and lipid composition. The four main types are ultra-low-density lipoprotein (ULDL), very-low-density lipoprotein (VLDL), low-density lipoprotein (LDL), intermediate-density lipoprotein (IDL) and high-density lipoprotein (HDL).

VLDL and IDL can convert to LDL, which is commonly known as "plaque". LDL contains the richest and purest cholesterol, as it has hardly any triglycerides. If too much of this waxy, whitish-yellow cholesterol accumulates in the arteries, it can block blood flow causing heart attack, stroke, or even death. To avoid this scenario, HDL helps to remove cholesterol from the bloodstream and artery walls and passes it on to the liver. Here cholesterol is processed and prepared for excretion from the body.

The Mediterranean style diet, known for its health benefits, can increase HDL levels. Virgin olive oil seems to play an important role here. On the other hand, "too much of a good thing" is not desirable, since high HDL levels increase the risk of heart disease. There's no reason to reduce or avoid using virgin olive oil, as excess HDL is more likely to be caused by smoking, alcohol, inflammation, type 2 diabetes, obesity, little or no physical activity, medications, the contraceptive pill, and estrogen replacement therapy. According to scientific findings, a balanced ratio between LDL and HDL and a healthy cholesterol level can prevent serious diseases.

The fact that cholesterol can compromise our health is only one side of the coin. The other side is that cholesterol is essential for the body as it builds the structure of cell membranes and forms sex hormones such as estrogens, progesterone, testosterone, and steroid hormones such as cortisol, aldosterone and adrenal hormones. It is involved in the formation of vitamin D and a component of bile salt. In fact, cholesterol is so important that the liver and intestines produce 80% of the body's requirement. The remaining 20 % is absorbed from food.

Women who have never had a problem with their cholesterol levels may be surprised to learn that this can change during menopause. Dr. Samia Mora, associate professor of medicine at Harvard Medical School and specialist in cardiovascular medicine in the Brigham and Women's Hospital, says this stage of life can put women into the risk group for heart disease. For this reason, it is important to keep an eye on cholesterol levels, especially during pre-menopause and the first few years after menopause. She also warns that factors specific to women are not sufficiently considered when calculating the estimated risk for heart attack and stroke. These include premature menopause (before the age of 40), pregnancy-related conditions such as preeclampsia, hypertension, gestational diabetes, and preterm birth. These conditions should be included in the screening because they can change a normal cholesterol level into a risk level. If you belong to the risk group but the standard test shows only normal levels, she recommends a coronary calcium scan and/or an apolipoprotein B blood test to make sure everything is really okay.

Do you feel constantly bloated and often full, even after a small meal or after waking up in the morning? Do you experience the need to burp regularly? What about unwanted weight loss, fatigue, and anemia? Or do you have a floating stool, perhaps clay-colored, that is difficult to flush down the toilet (steatorrhea)? These are all signs that you are having trouble digesting fats properly because the digestion and absorption process is compromised. There are several reasons why this can happen. Fat malabsorption may be the result of gastric resection or radiation-induced injuries, and pancreatic enzyme dysfunction, which is often a first sign of celiac disease. Other causes include infections, dysfunctional microbiome, lymphatic system, circulation, and enzymes of the small intestine, which are responsible for motility and removal of intestinal gases. If these enzymes do not function properly, they can increase intestinal hypersensitivity and rectal distension. A rare but possible cause is the hereditary disease chylomicronemia, in which fat particles accumulate in the blood because of inadequate metabolism.

Dietary fat intake often worsens symptoms of IBS. The cause could be a bile acid malabsorption (BAM), sometimes called bile acid diarrhea (BAD). Symptoms include watery stools, urinary urgency, and fecal incontinence. The liver releases bile acids, especially during high-fat meals, which slowly enter the small intestine to aid digestion. Usually, these bile acids are reabsorbed and returned to the liver, where they await the next meal. If these bile acids cannot be absorbed properly, the production of bile is stimulated. The excess bile acid is forced to flow through the large intestine instead of returning to the liver, adding more water to this organ, which in turn causes diarrhea. According to research, one-third of IBS-D patients suffer from BAM, but so do 50% of people with functional diarrhea and 35% of people with microscopic colitis or inflammatory bowel diseases such as celiac disease and Crohn's disease.

It is not easy to diagnose BAM because the testing options are limited. There are two tests available in the U.S. - the serum 7αC4 test and the fecal bile acid test. Europe and Canada offer a third - the SeHCAT test. In the past, tests were done with bile secretion agents, but these treatments are often not well tolerated, especially formulations with resin such as cholestyramine, according to Dr. Michael Camilleri, a gastroenterologist at the Mayo Clinic in Minnesota.

Any signs of fat malabsorption - and other nutrient malabsorption - should be discussed with your doctor, as you may have a serious underlying condition such as celiac disease, Crohn's disease, chronic pancreatitis, or cystic fibrosis.

Over the course of my life, I have witnessed directly how the nutrition world has changed from advocating low-fat diets to high-fat diets. What was initially demonized is now touted as beneficial. While fat can be beneficial to our cells, there is little point in eating a lot of it if you have problems with fat malabsorption. I wish I had known earlier that fat can be problematic in gastrointestinal disorders, because I often wondered why I didn't feel better during a particular diet. I blamed many foods, but fat was never one of them. Reducing my fat consumption, especially coconut oil and ghee, made a big difference. These days I use different oils and fats sparingly.

## SATURATED FAT

We all need some fat in our diet to keep our body functioning. However, not all fats are the same. In general, all fats consist of carbon, hydrogen, and oxygen, but differ in their chemical bonds. When a fat is densely packed with hydrogen molecules, it is called a "saturated fat". It is usually solid at room temperature. While a looser chemical bond makes a fat an "unsaturated fat" with a more liquid consistency. Although it seems like a small difference, it can affect our health in one way or another.

When you search the internet, you'll find controversial information about saturated fat. Even scientists don't quite agree on whether saturated fat is bad for us or not. But what we know is that saturated fat is associated with the raise of LDL cholesterol levels in the blood which can lead to an increased risk of heart attack and stroke. For the prevention of these diseases, it is recommended to reduce the intake of saturated fats and replace it with polyunsaturated fats - a type of unsaturated fat, which I will come to later. This approach is more easily said than done, because saturated fat is very common in the modern standard diet. It comes mainly from animals and is therefore found in red meat, lard, and dairy products such as butter, cream and ghee. It is a well-used ingredient in the food industry. Snacks, baked goods, convenience foods, you name it, it's in it. Even if you are vegetarian or vegan you will find saturated fat in plant foods, such as the kernel of the *Cocos nucifera* and the *Elaeis guineensis* palms - coconut oil and palm kernel oil.

In recent years, coconut oil has been hyped up as a "miracle food" that supposedly boosts the immune system, supports weight loss, regulates blood sugar levels, promotes brain function and heart health. As the name implies, coconut oil is extracted from the fruit of the coconut palm, which is abundant in tropical and subtropical regions of the world. Countries like Indonesia, the Philippines and India are the world's leading producers of this oil. Due to its long history and extensive use in these cuisines, the digestive systems of the people in these regions have adapted well to this difficult-to-digest oil. This is not necessarily the case for people in the West.

Coconut oil has a high energy density and is about 90% saturated fat. One tablespoon provides 117 kcal (489 kJ) but unlike olive oil, it hardly provides any micronutrients such as vitamins and minerals. One reason coconut oil is so popular today is that researchers say it is less harmful than other saturated fats as it contains the medium-chain triglycerides (MCTs). MCT promote weight loss, reduce waist circumference, convert ketones (keto diet!) into energy when carbohydrate intake is low, and can increase the beneficial HDL cholesterol. However, coconut oil contains not only MCTs, but also a large amount of lauric acid, which is difficult to absorb in the small intestine. The reason for this shortcoming is that lauric acid is a medium-chain fatty acid that behaves like a long-chain fatty acid during digestion. If you already have problems with the small intestine, it may be a better idea to use an MTC oil or powder rather than taking coconut oil by the spoonful.

MTC oil is an odorless and colorless liquid that is easier to digest than coconut oil because it does not require enzymes or bile acids to break it down. It is manufactured by extracting (fractionating) caprylic acid and capric acid from coconut or palm kernel oil. Both acids are blended to produce MCT oil. Some people experience digestive problems consuming the pure oil but may have less problems with the MCT powder. The powder is convenient because you can take it with you without making an oily mess. You can use it as a coffee creamer or for giving a smoothie a nice texture. This powder is made from spray-dried MCT oil mixed with a little starch. This process reduces the MCT oil content. The ratio of starch to oil can vary greatly from product to product. Some people experience health issues when consuming these powders, which is probably due to the fact that the starch may have come from corn, dairy, or grains - corn fiber, sodium caseinate, or maltodextrin. To avoid digestive or allergy problems, look for a product that is made from 100% coconut - not a blend of coconut and palm oil – and is free of additives, thickeners, and emulsifiers. It should contain only medium-chain triglycerides and a binder such as acacia fiber.

Of course, if you want to use real coconut oil, you have the choice between refined and unrefined products. Usually, refined coconut oil is made of dried coconut "meat", also called copra, pressed through a machine, heated, and filtered. During this process, chemicals may be used to remove all impurities and bacteria. The disadvantage of this method is that the copra undergoes a long drying process in humid tropical conditions, with the risk that it will develop mold. In addition, some of these coconut oil products are hydrogenated or partially hydrogenated to extend their shelf-life. During the manufacturing process these products are partially transformed into trans-fats, a specific type of unsaturated fat that has several negative health effects. Refined coconut oil is tasteless and odorless. It has a high smoke point of up to 459°F (232°C). The temperature is measure of how hot a cooking fat can be heated before it burns, produces smoke, and releases harmful chemicals.

An unrefined oil such as virgin coconut oil, expeller-pressed coconut oil or cold-pressed coconut oil is made from fresh coconut meat, but is also more expensive. The first two unrefined oils are produced with a small amount of heat or steam, while the cold-pressed coconut oil is not. Unrefined oils have a much lower smoking point of 350°F (177°C) and are therefore not suitable for use with high temperatures, such as deep frying.

Coconut oil is a powerful antimicrobial agent that does not distinguish between beneficial and undesirable bacteria in its action. Its weapons against bacteria are MCFAs. These MCFAs are usually absorbed via the portal vein, but sometimes also through the intestine. When the MCFAs in the intestines destroy gram-negative bacteria, fragments of the outer cell wall of the bacteria, known as endotoxins or LPS, can be released. The remaining MCFA and LPS can be incorporated into chylomicrons and enter the bloodstream initiating an immune response. Through the union with chylomicrons, LPS can enter the bloodstream initiating an immune response and may cause inflammation, infection, fever, or even a septic shock. In a healthy individual, LPS do not pose a threat; rather, they are part of a resilient immune response. This might not be true for everyone as a study on mice shows that after an injection with LPS, a transient inflammatory response occurred in the small intestine, resulting in tissue damage. People with a weak immune system, such as newborns, the elderly, and the chronically ill, have a much higher risk of developing severe complications from this endotoxin. If you have an impaired gastrointestinal tract or an overgrowth of bacteria in the intestine, it may be a good idea to use coconut oil sparingly to avoid an increase of endotoxin in the blood.

## UNSATURATED FAT

Unsaturated fats have many health benefits. For example, they lower LDL cholesterol levels while maintaining HDL cholesterol levels, improve blood vessel function, and may even have a positive effect on insulin levels and blood sugar control, which is particularly important for people with type 2 diabetes. As with any fat, it is recommended to consume them in moderation as they are high in calories. Unsaturated fats should be used instead of saturated fat, not in addition to them. It's also wise to cut back on carbohydrate-rich foods if you're eating more fats. This can help with weight loss.

It is not easy to navigate through the complex world of unsaturated fats, with its MUFAs and PUFAs, omegas and alphas, EPAs, and DHAs, but doing so can lead to a better understanding of what is good for you. Unsaturated fats are mainly divided into two groups: monounsaturated fatty acids (MUFAs) and polyunsaturated fatty acids (PUFAs), which differ slightly in their chemical structure. MUFAs have a single carbon-to-carbon double bond, whereas PUFAs have two or more of these bonds. These bonds are the reason for their behavior at certain temperatures. The type of unsaturated fat determines the respective smoke point. For example, avocado oil can be heated up to 520°F (271°C), while flaxseed oil is much too delicate to be heated at all. Many unsaturated oils are used only as finishing oils to enhance dishes or as a salad dressing.

MUFAs are liquid at room temperature and semi-solid or solid when chilled. They come from animal and plant sources. MUFAs are particularly health-promoting when derived from a plant source as they help to decrease the risk of developing cardiovascular disease and type 2 diabetes. MUFAs from animal products such as red meat and dairy products provide no benefits. Beneficial MUFAs are highly represented in the Mediterranean style diet with foods such as olive oil, peanut oil, canola oil, nuts, avocados, olives, seeds, whole grain, and fatty fish including salmon and mackerel. Note that these cooking oils can become bitter if heated too much.

PUFAs contain *essential* fatty acids that the body cannot synthesize and therefore must be supplied through diet. They are needed for cell membranes and the coating of nerves, for the blood clotting process, muscle movement and during inflammation. PUFA is a type of fat that is mainly in vegetable oils such as sunflower, safflower, sesame, soybean, and corn oil. When heated above 175°F (80°C) these oils begin to oxidize, and when ingested, cause stress to the body and can lead to inflammation. PUFAs are vulnerable not only to heat, but also to light and oxygen. In other words: if a clear bottle of oil sits on the supermarket shelf for months, it can turn into an oil of concern. The same applies to the more fragile PUFA oils such as flaxseed oil, sesame oil, walnut oil, and fish oil - even though they are normally not heated. They require special attention as they can easily become rancid if not kept in a dark bottle and in the refrigerator.

There are two well-known types of PUFAs – omega-3 and omega-6. The term omega and the appended number stand for a specific position in the chemical structure of the polyunsaturated fat. Both types are converted into hormones and act in every cell and tissue of the body. They are rich in vitamin E, which is an important antioxidant that can remove harmful substances (oxalates) from the body. It is desirable to find the right balance between the pro-inflammatory omega-6 and the anti-inflammatory omega-3 fatty acids in our diet. This may be easier said than done, since omega-6 is abundant in our diet, while omega-3 is not. In the average Western diet, the balance between these PUFAs has become out of whack. Instead of the evolutionary equal ratio of 1:1, it is now 20:1 in favor of omega-6. Many people are not aware of how much omega-6 they are consuming, as almost all plant seeds and grains contain this substance. The exception is seeds from coconut, cocoa, and palm trees. As vegetable oil is an essential ingredient in many processed foods such as cookies, cakes and takeaway meals, these foods also contain omega-6. Even if you eat meat, you are consuming this PUFA, because the livestock feed is often grain.

In comparison, omega-3 foods such as fatty fish, flaxseed, walnut, or hydrogenated soybean oils do not find their way into our kitchens as easily. They are more perishable due to environmental influences. In addition, the lack of omega-3 fatty acids may be due to the fact that the enzymes responsible for converting PUFAs cannot distinguish between omega-3 and omega-6 fatty acids. The motto is first come, first served - which means that omega-6 has a great chance of winning the race because we consume so much more of it. When omega-6 is prevalent in our bodies it causes inflammation in the tissues and promotes diseases such as atherosclerosis, obesity, and diabetes. The remedy is to consume less omega-6 and more omega-3 as it helps to reduce inflammation and strengthens lymphatic functions, which in turn benefits the gastrointestinal system.

To better understand omega-3, we need to look at the subdivision of this fatty acid. There are three types of omega-3: eicosapentaenoic acid (EPA), alpha-linolenic acid (ALA), and docosahexaenoic acid (DHA). The latter is primarily needed in the cerebral cortex, brain, retina, testes, and sperm. Fatty fish such as wild Atlantic salmon, mackerel, and swordfish are good sources of EPA and DHA. To get enough of them, you can eat oily fish once or twice a week. Or, if you don't like fish or are vegan, you could include algae foods such as kelp, dulse, spirulina, and chlorella in your diet, although they contain far less omega-3 acid than the fish. If you regularly eat green leafy vegetables and use oils made from flaxseed, canola, chia, perilla, or walnuts, you will get a good amount of ALA. To some extent, the body can convert ALA into DHA and EPA, but this may not always be enough for its need. Researchers found that milk from grass-fed cows has a much better balance of omega-6 and omega-3 than that from conventionally and organically farmed cows with little or no access to pasture. Watch out for the unregulated term "grass-fed" on packages, as it can be misleading. This term is often used when cattle are only occasionally allowed to graze on pastures. Otherwise, they are fed grains that can be of organic or conventional origin. True "grass-fed" animals eat only grass for their entire lives, nothing else!

Many people try to meet their need for EPA and DHA by taking fish oil because it is praised in the media or recommended by their healthcare providers. It is controversial whether fish oil is beneficial, harmful, or even ineffective. Marketing claims that it can prevent cancer or other serious diseases, but this promise should be taken with a grain of salt. Chris Kresser says in one of his blog posts (March 17, 2019), that EPA and DHA are susceptible to oxidation from light, oxygen, and heat. Due to manufacturing, many of the over-the-counter fish oil supplements are highly oxidized and can pose a health risk including organ toxicity and accelerated atherosclerosis. He goes on to say that these supplements often do not have the EPA and DHA levels stated on the bottle. Besides, they may not be as effective as eating the real thing – fish!

If you opt for the fish, be sure that it contains as little mercury as possible. The accumulation of this substance in the body can lead to poisoning. The Australian government offers a list that features fish high in omega-3 and low in mercury, which includes herring, sardine, mackerel, silver warehou, and Atlantic salmon. Other fish that are low in mercury, but contain less omega-3, are snapper, whiting, mullet, bream, trevally, garfish, squid, and trout. From a health (not environmental) point of view, wild fish are preferable because they feed on microalgae, unlike farmed fish, which are fed all kinds of things and may not necessarily be kept in a species-appropriate manner. Chris Kresser also points out that the ALA from flax, hemp, pumpkin seeds, and walnuts may not produce enough DHA due to their biochemical limitations. He recommends vegetarians and vegans supplement with microalgae daily to avoid nutrient deficiencies.

## TRANS-FATS

The worst dietary fat is trans-fat, an unhealthy unsaturated fat. It is a product of the food industry that converts liquid fat into solid fat, like shorting or margarine, to prevent it from going rancid. Even small amounts of trans-fat can become harmful, as it can raise LDL, lower HDL and cause cholesterol to build up in the blood vessels, inflammation, type 2 diabetes, and heart diseases. Some governments have banned trans-fats in their countries because of their health risk, but many only enact regulations to limit their use in food production. Since this fat is so convenient for the food industry, companies still find ways to smuggle it into their products. The National Heart Foundation of Australia report (2017), disappointingly shows that there has been no evidence of a significant decrease in the use of trans-fats over the past 15 years. The problem has only shifted. Trans-fats may no longer be in our margarine, but it is now in meat pies, pastries, sausages rolls, popcorn, scones, doughnuts, dry pasta, takeaways. In fact, anything cooked in oil at extremely high temperatures, such as fried foods, contains this unhealthy fat. Pay special attention when you see the words "hydrogenated" or "partially hydrogenated" fat or oil in the ingredients list on the product label. Both are synonyms for trans-fats.

# DIETARY FIBER

Perhaps you have heard from your parents or grandparents that you should eat more vegetables? Or a doctor may have advised you to eat more dietary fiber to keep your bowel movements going. They may have recommended that you use one of those fiber powders from the pharmacy. You may have had an unpleasant experience after eating much more fiber than you normally would. Now you may be wondering what the fiber is all about.

First and foremost, fiber is magic! It melts excess pounds from the body, and by pulling a few extra tricks out of its sleeve, it banishes diseases and prolongs our lives. Anyone can become a magician by eating enough high-fiber foods such as fruits, vegetables, nuts, seeds, whole grains, and legumes. Refined and processed foods, including canned fruits and vegetables, juices without pulp, white breads, pasta, and rice, virtually all foods containing hulled grains, provide little or no dietary fiber. If we take a closer look at its tricks, the indigestible fibrous parts pass unhindered through the small intestine and are transported to the large intestine, where they solidify feces. This results in mechanical stimulation of peristalsis, which in turn promotes increased secretion to enhance elimination. Bacteria contribute to this process by feeding on this fibrous material, making dietary fiber a prebiotic.

There are even more surprises to fiber, as it also has anti-inflammatory properties and helps release the hormone insulin, which is produced by the pancreas to keep blood sugar levels in balance. This makes dietary fiber an invaluable aid in the prevention of type 2 diabetes. If that wasn't enough, researchers found that a high-fiber diet and a reduction in animal protein reduces waist circumference and prolongs one's life. The latter finding is related to the fact that dietary fiber can positively influence the length of telomeres – a specific structure at the end of our DNA. Telomeres have a protective function as they can delay or even reverse the cellular aging process. They are a bit like the plastic caps on shoelaces. When these caps break, the lace frays and is no longer usable. The same principle applies to telomeres and DNA. Due to aging or other reasons, telomeres shrink and are of limited use for cellular functions, leading to defective cells that can cause inflammation or even cancer. The good news is that regular consumption of dietary fiber can protect or even restore the length of telomeres. Longer telomeres are a sign of slow aging and a decline in diseases such as cardiovascular disease, cancer, Alzheimer's and Parkinson's. Given all these wonderful health benefits, it's quite surprising that so many people don't pay enough attention to their daily fiber intake.

With SIBO and IBS, you may have difficulty including dietary fiber into your diet as you experience symptoms such as bloating, gas, constipation, abdominal discomfort, and pain. Dr. Will Bulsiewicz, a gastroenterologist, author of *Fiber Fueled. The Plant-Based Gut Health Program for Losing Weight, Restoring Your Health, and Optimizing Your Microbiome*, and creator of the Dr. B website, urges us not to lose sight of fiber as it is so important to our health. In his professional career and through personal experience, he saw firsthand the power of fiber and the positive effects it has on IBS, leaky gut and other digestive issues. The long-term goal should be to include as much fiber as possible into your diet. That said, many people change their diet too much or too quickly when they introduce a new approach into their lives. In terms of dietary fiber, it is strongly recommended to increase your intake only gradually, that is by no more than 0.18 oz (5 g) per day per week. This allows the microbiome to adjust to this dietary change. Drink plenty of water throughout the day to soften the stool and make it easier to pass.

Not all types of fiber are beneficial to conditions such as SIBO and IBS, as they can contain high levels of FODMAPs. According to Australia's Monash University, dietary fiber is usually not responsible for discomfort, but rather its FODMAP content is. The difference between FODMAPs and dietary fiber lies in the fermentation process, with the latter being digested in a slower and more controlled manner compared to FODMAPs. Suitable dietary fibers for SIBO and IBS have a medium viscosity, are soluble and moderately fermentable, for example oats (beta-glucans), barley, psyllium, and raw guar gum. A dietary supplement with these properties may be of particular benefit in all forms of IBS (IBS-D, IBS-M, and IBS-C) when consumption of fresh foods causes problems.

Dietary fiber is classified into the following groups according to its degradability in the large intestine: soluble dietary fibers, insoluble dietary fibers, and resistant starch. Let's go through them all and see what benefits and drawbacks they might have for a compromised small intestine.

## SOLUBLE FIBER

Soluble fibers are dispersible in water, form a gel-like consistency, and are metabolized by the inhabitants of the large intestine. During this fermentation process, SCFAs such as acetate, propionate, and butyrate are produced and gases are released. It's quite amazing, because this SCFA production provides around 10% of our daily requirements. A lack of soluble fiber in our diet can cause an impaired microbiome due to an imbalance between its inhabitants and the virtual disappearance of certain beneficial bacterial strains. Such a situation in the gut can increase the risk of developing inflammatory bowel disease, multiple sclerosis, diabetes, allergies, asthma, autism and cancer. A regular consumption of soluble fiber keeps the microbial community happy, maintains blood sugar levels, supports heart health, and prevents con-stipation – which means less pressure in the intestine and therefore less abdominal pain. Soluble fiber cannot be lumped together as there are many different types, including inulin, polydextrose, psyllium, gum, pectin, beta-glucans, and wheat dextrin. The different types of soluble fiber have different properties.

Inulin, also called long-chain inulin, an indigestible oligo, is a natural component of plants. This highly fermentable dietary fiber can help in various gastrointestinal diseases by stimulating the growth of beneficial bacteria in the large intestine such as *Bifidobacterium* and *Lactobacillus*. This fiber acts as a prebiotic. Consumption may not be very wise if you have an overgrowth of bacteria in your small intestine, as it may then ferment in the wrong place. Depending on the severity of the disease, it must be weighed whether this fiber should be eliminated from the diet for a certain period or not. This might not an easy task as there are many foods that contain large amounts of inulin. Vegetables include chicory, Jerusalem artichoke, dandelion, asparagus, onion, garlic, leek, shallots, beets, fennel, cabbage, green peas, snow peas, and sweetcorn. Fruits include custard apples, nectarines, white peaches, watermelon, grapefruit, pomegranate, green/unripe bananas, and dried fruits such as dates and figs. Inulin is also found in chickpeas, lentils, red kidney beans, soybeans, cashew, pistachios, wheat, rye, barley, and oats.

Inulin is not limited to fresh products, as derived sugar extracts are also found in processed foods. For manufacturers, these extracts are a popular and cost-effective way to increase the dietary fiber content of their products to make them more attractive to consumers. Due to current dietary trends, inulin is mainly added to products labeled as "high-fiber", "gluten-free", "dairy-free" and "low-fat". It gives these products a slightly sweet taste, a creamier texture, and mimics the elasticity of gluten. However, it is also found in other products such as candy bars, drinks, ice cream, infant formula, protein shakes, muffins, energy bars, rice-based breakfast cereals, scones, breads, cottage and cream cheese.

If you check the product packaging, you will find many different names for inulin such as chicory root extract or fiber, fructo-oligos, neosugar, alant, starch, alant starch, alantin, dahlin and diabetic sugar. Although the inulin agents are supposedly safe, and even suitable for diabetics, they can have an adverse effect on an already disturbed digestive system. For example, they increase gas production in the gut and thus contribute to flatulence, bloating, cramps, abdominal pain, diarrhea, and sometimes even constipation. This gas-forming property is also present in the soluble dietary fiber of polydextrose - dextrose, sorbitol, and citric acid - a sugar substitute and filler used often in processed foods.

If you want to avoid fermentation in the small intestine and need support for constipation or diarrhea, the soluble fiber psyllium may be the right choice for you. But don't take my word for it, because for some people symptoms may actually get worse, or they experience no change at all. Psyllium is extracted from the plant *Plantago ovata*, native to parts of Asia, the Mediterranean region, and North Africa. Psyllium is particularly useful in reducing bloating and as a laxative. It has wound healing properties and removes bacteria, worms, and toxins from the digestive tract. In cases of diarrhea or fecal incontinence, it helps to firm fecal matter. Aside from its fecal merits, psyllium, like the beta-glucan found in oats, can help lower LDL cholesterol and blood sugar levels. One study discovered its weight-controlling properties. The researchers observed that their test group taking psyllium lost an average of 7.2 pounds (3.3 kg) of their original weight after six months of use. The control group, which took the soluble fiber guar gum, lost only half as much weight. Psyllium can also be used to maintain remission in inflammatory bowel diseases such as ulcerative colitis and Crohn's disease, but again, the results are very variable.

Psyllium can be purchased in the form of capsules, tablets, wafers, husks, and seeds in health food stores, pharmacies, or even some super-markets. A well-known brand of laxative that contains psyllium is Metamucil. I personally prefer to buy psyllium in the health-food store as a husk to avoid additional ingredients such as flavors, colors, and sugars. If you use a commercial product, please follow the instructions on the label. If you use a loose product such as psyllium husk, mix it with plenty of warm water before drinking. It forms a viscous gel that takes some getting used to when swallowed. Start with a small daily dose of psyllium husk, for example half a teaspoon in about 8 oz (230 ml) of water and drink it before a meal, such as breakfast or dinner. After about a week, you can increase the dose as needed by taking it twice a day. If you tolerate this amount and feel well the following week, you can continue to increase the intake – up to two teaspoons per dose. As a rule, you should avoid excessive consumption and always drink plenty of water throughout the day, otherwise symptoms such as constipation and swelling may occur. If drinking psyllium gel water doesn't appeal to you, you can sprinkle the husk or powder on your breakfast cereal, or cook and bake with it. I add a tablespoon of psyllium husk to my homemade gluten-free baked goods to give them extra fiber and a bread-like texture.

Keep in mind, psyllium can interact with medications. It is advisable to talk to your doctor before adding it into your diet. Sometime only a small adjustment in dosage or timing is needed to avoid problems. Special care should also be taken if you suffer from conditions such as intestinal cramps, difficulty swallowing, narrowing or obstructions of the gastrointestinal tract. Children should consult a doctor before taking psyllium supplements. For them, as for adults, it is important that they get their fiber primarily from whole foods rather than from a supplement.

Gum is another type of soluble fiber found in the sap of almost all plants, that is, in the stems, branches, and fruits. Gum is a sticky substance that becomes completely soluble or soft in water, forming a thick, sticky liquid or slime that is usually odorless and tasteless. Chris Kresser notes that gums are generally not harmful, but people with digestive problems may experience intolerances. Given this likelihood, he recommends avoiding certain gums known to have these effects at the start of your health journey.

For example, there is the refined food-grade carrageenan. It is added to non-dairy products such as almond milk and coconut milk. It can harm the intestine by damaging epithelial cells, increasing the risk of leaky gut and inflammation. This food-grade carrageenan should not be confused with degraded carrageenan, also known as poligeenan. Poligeenan has been shown to be carcinogenic in animal studies. However, it is not used in the food industry.

Guar gum is a gluten-free whitish powder extracted from the guar bean (also known as gavar, gawar or guvar bean), which grows mainly in India and Pakistan. The peculiarity of this gum is that it slows the growth of ice crystals, which is particularly convenient for frozen products, as they remain stable for longer periods outside the freezer. The use of guar gum is not limited to these frozen products as it is also a popular stabilizer in cottage cheese, yogurt, sauces, and soups. Researchers found that the consumption of foods that are enhanced with guar gum can be effective for weight loss, to reduce blood sugar levels and total cholesterol. Chris Kresser advises against using guar gum initially for IBS and SIBO because it can increase bloating and abdominal discomfort. A similar problem arises with the locust bean gum, also known as carob bean. You may want to reintroduce these gums at a later stage of your treatment and see if you can tolerate them then.

Xanthan gum is a popular food additive and is often used as a thickener or stabilizer to improve the texture of products, for example to give elasticity to gluten-free products. In Australia and New Zealand, it is hidden behind the number E415. Xanthan gum differs from other gums in that it is not derived from a plant. It is formed during the fermentation of sugar by a bacterium called *Xanthomonas campestris*. People with food allergies, intolerances and celiac disease should avoid this product because the culture medium in which these bacteria grow is soy, wheat, corn, or dairy. There is a likelihood that protein residues from the culture medium will enter the final product during the manufacturing process. Since it is a fermented product, it could affect someone who is hypersensitive to mold. Vegans should also be vigilant, as not all xanthan gum is free of animal products. Since there is no detailed information on the product packaging about the manufacturing process, Chris Kresser recommends avoiding xanthan gum if you belong to any of the above groups. It is not easy to get around this popular ingredient, as it is widely used in ice cream, salad dressings, puddings, yogurt, sauces, frozen foods, beverages, low-fat foods, gluten-free foods, and even pharmaceutical products. Xanthan gum is also found in non-food products such as toothpaste, cosmetics, oven and toilet cleaner, adhesives like wallpaper glue, paints, fungicides, herbicides, and insecticides. Animal studies, and in the few human studies, show that xanthan gum increases bile acid, resulting in a softer and larger stool volume, making it a potential laxative. It lowers serum sugar levels, increases the amount of SCFAs - keeping the microbiome healthy – and to Chris Kresser's surprise, it has antitumor properties that help slow melanoma cancer in mice. The side effect of this gum is an increased production of hydrogen gas, bloating, and diarrhea symptoms. If you consume large amounts - more than 0.5 oz (15 g) per day - you may also experience stomach upset.

Xanthan gum should not be given to infants, as their intestinal tracts are not yet mature and may not be able to handle an increase in SCFA. You can replace xanthan gum with arrowroot flour in cooking, as it has a similar effect in baking and sauces. Arrowroot is a starchy root vegetable related to yam, cassava, and taro. It a well-known, old-fashioned remedy for diarrhea, but it also provides nutrition and a soothing action on intestinal tissues. When consumed, 20% passes through the small intestine and enters the large intestine where it is metabolized by bacteria. If the small intestine is overpopulated with bacteria, consumption should be avoided for some time until your condition has improved.

The sap of the thorny *Acacia senegal* tree gushes from its branches and is processed into arabic gum, also called gum arabic, sudani, senegal gum and India gum. It is a popular ingredient in the food industry and commonly used in ice cream, chilled desserts, fillings, soft drinks, chewing gum, and candy. Like many of the other gums, it usually passes harmlessly through the small intestine unless there is a digestive disorder. It acts as a prebiotic. Researchers found that arabic gum supplementation of 0.4 oz (10 g) per day significantly increased the population of *Bifidobacterium* and *Lactobacillus* strains within four weeks. A dose of up to 1 oz (30 g) may be well tolerated but may cause excessive bloating when first taken. Other side effects include mild diarrhea and morning nausea. As with the consumption of most gums, it is possible for inflammation to worsen in the gastrointestinal tract. If you do not notice an increase in symptoms, you can continue taking it. Arabic gum significantly reduced the body mass index and body fat in a healthy female research group, according to a double-blind study. It also has an antioxidant effect and offers some protection against liver and heart toxicity. In Sudan, where most arabic gum comes from, it is prescribed to patients with chronic kidney failure because it improves their lives by reducing the frequency of dialysis. Due to a lack of research, Chris Kresser recommends avoiding tara and gellan gums. It might be a good idea to avoid them in the meantime until more human studies have been done.

Pectin is another wonderful soluble dietary fiber, also known as modified citrus pectin (MCP). It is in many fruits, vegetables, legumes, nuts, and seeds and especially abundant in carrots, apples and citrus fruits - including their seeds. In manufactured foods, pectin is commonly used as an emulsifier, stabilizer, thickener, gelling agent, as well as a sugar substitute in low-calorie foods. Dentists know it as an adhesive for dentures. Pectin has all the health benefits that other soluble fiber has, and in addition, it can significantly improve stool formation in IBS-D.

Some people experience an allergic reaction when they eat common fruits such as apples, peaches, sugar melons, kiwis, cherries, grapes, strawberries, bananas, pudding apples, mangoes, and pomegranates. These severe symptoms usually appear a few minutes after consumption and can manifest as itching and swelling of the mouth, lungs, face, nose, and stomach. Other people do not tolerate these foods well, possibly due to their content of FODMAPs, and experience digestive issues. When chemical exposure from modern agriculture is added to these conditions, things can get even worse. It is best to eat organically grown fruits and vegetables wherever you can. Every year, the nonprofit Environmental Working Group publishes a "dirty dozen" list of the most chemically sprayed agricultural products. High levels of pesticides are currently found on strawberries, spinach, kale, nectarines, and apples, followed by grapes, peaches, cherries, pears, tomatoes, celery, and potatoes.

Apples are a popular ingredient in Ayurvedic cooking. It is said that eating stewed apples in combination with spices early in the morning awakens a healthy appetite for lunch, which according to their tradition is the most important meal of the day. This dish helps to ignite a "digestive fire" that promotes the production of healthy gastric juices and digestive enzymes. At the same time, it is said to increase vitality, stimulate bowel movement, and prevent constipation. Numerous studies praise the benefits of the apple for its richness in micronutrients (polyphenols), which are contained mainly in its peel. There are over a thousand different polyphenols, not all of which have yet been recorded. It seems that polyphenols are a "lucky bag" of antioxidant and anti-inflammatory properties that help to prevent many diseases such as cardiovascular diseases, neurodegenerative disorders, cancer, and obesity.

Dietary fiber creates a relationship with polyphenols. Researchers say dietary fiber controls the accessibility of polyphenols in the gut by influencing bacteria responsible for polyphenol metabolism, to such an extent that some fiber-containing foods may even inhibit the release of polyphenols in the upper part of the digestive tract, benefiting the lower part of the intestine. On the other hand, polyphenols can influence the fermentation of dietary fiber, as some types have both antibacterial and prebiotic properties.

Apples are not the only food with high polyphenol content. Other foods include berries, plums, sweet cherries, blackcurrants, black and white beans, vegetables such as artichokes, chicory, red onions and spinach and nuts such as hazelnuts, almonds, walnuts, and pecans. It is also found in soya products, black and green tea, cocoa powder, dark chocolate, red wine, and spices such as cloves. Excessive consumption of polyphenol supplements should be avoided, as they can have a negative impact on health. In large quantities, this substance interferes with iron absorption and causes thyroid problems as well as a change in estrogen levels. Interactions with prescription drugs are also possible.

One of my favorite foods is homemade, unsweetened applesauce made from organic apples. It's a great source of fiber, minerals and vitamins. It's so easy to make that I don't even peel the apples because I want to keep all the goodies. I just wash them, remove the core and cut them into big pieces. Then I boil them with a little water and maybe add a stick or two of cinnamon, which has anti-fungal, anti-microbial and anti-inflammatory properties. Cinnamon also helps with diarrhea and strengthens the intestines. After the apples have simmered on low for a while, I remove the cinnamon sticks and puree the apples. The applesauce keeps well in the refrigerator, but for better digestion I reheat it before eating.

Next in the line of soluble fiber comes beta-glucan. It is found mainly in the cell walls of bacteria and also in fungi, yeast, algae, lichen, raw guar gum, mushrooms, and plants such as oats and barley. Food manufacturers use beta-glucan as an additive in products such as salad dressings, frozen desserts, sour cream, and cheese spreads. It may also be found in dietary supplements and medications. The efficacy of beta-glucan in terms of lowering blood sugar, total cholesterol, and blood lipid profile has been extensively studied. It plays a role in weight loss and is recognized as an inti-inflammatory and immunomodulator with antitumor activity. It is safe to use for most people, but because it simulates the immune system, those with autoimmune diseases such as multiple sclerosis, lupus, rheumatoid arthritis, asthma, and inflammatory bowel disease should be especially careful. We do not yet have enough information on how it affects these diseases.

The non-viscous soluble dietary fiber wheat dextrin is derived from wheat starch and used to increase the fiber content in many processed foods. It is also found in dietary supplements. It has no water-binding capacity and is therefore not suitable as a laxative. Rather, it tends to cause constipation when taken in doses greater than 0.4 oz (10 g) per day. Like inulin, wheat dextrin helps to lower LDL and total cholesterol as well as blood sugar levels. People with celiac disease or gluten sensitivity should not take this fiber as it may contain gluten. Check the information on the label before consuming this product.

## INSOLUBLE FIBER

Plant foods generally contain fiber in the ratio one-third soluble and two-thirds insoluble fiber. Insoluble fiber is the structural part of plant cell walls and, unlike soluble fiber, does not dissolve in water or form a gel. The fermentation capacity is quite limited. All insoluble fiber contributes to the compactness of the stool and acceleration of motility. Due to this fact it can prevent constipation and diverticular disease. This disease is known for its pockets in the intestinal wall, where microorganisms can colonize and cause inflammation. Its symptoms include bloating, abdominal pain, fever, nausea, vomiting, abdominal tenderness, mucus in the stool, and a change in bowel habits such as constipation or diarrhea. There are many foods including fruits and vegetable peels, legumes, whole grains, nuts, seeds and bran from wheat and rice that contain insoluble fiber. Coarse insoluble fiber particles can irritate intestinal tissues, leading to increased water retention and diarrhea. Common types of insoluble fiber are lignin, cellulose, and some hemicelluloses.

Lignin is considered a non-carbohydrate form of fiber that is completely indigestible and poorly metabolized by intestinal bacteria. It is found in woody plants and in the husk of grains. Other foods include bitter melon (bitter gourd), beans, peas, green plantain, apples, kiwifruit, linseeds, edible seeds - from berries and tomatoes - and root vegetables such as parsnip, carrots, horseradish, and beetroots, as well as edible stems such as those from parsley, broccoli and cabbage.

Cellulose provides structure and strength to the cell walls of plants, and like lignin, is poorly metabolized by intestinal bacteria. It is found in wheat and rice bran, legumes, root vegetables, apple skins, collard greens, and kale. When industrially modified, the natural cellulose becomes water-soluble. This newly formed ingredient is used as an additive in processed foods. Since the effects of natural and modified cellulose on humans have not yet been sufficiently researched, only limited information about this fiber is available.

Hemicelluloses are a group of structures that occur in the plant cell wall. One of these is arabinoxylan that can be found in psyllium, flaxseed, bamboo shoots, grasses and grains such as rye, wheat, barley, corn, oats, millet, rice, sorghum. Hemicelluloses are also used in the food industry as thickeners, stabilizers, emulsifiers, and additives. They can be a component of prebiotic supplements. Their high water-binding capacity promotes faster passage of waste products from the intestine. A small double-blind study showed that a modified arabinoxylan from rice bran (Biobran) led to a significant improvement of IBS symptoms. Other researchers emphasize that arabinoxylan-enriched foods can lower blood sugar and triglyceride levels – though they can cause diarrhea, bloating, and stomach pain in some people.

## RESISTANT STARCH

A unique insoluble fiber is resistant starch. As its name implies, this food resists digestion in the small intestine and passes almost untouched into the large intestine, where it is metabolized by bacteria. Resistant starch is found in foods such as beans, legumes, starchy fruits and vegetables, whole grains, nuts, tiger nuts - which are tubers rather than nuts - and particularly in uncooked, non-rolled oats. Cooked and cooled potato and rice dishes are also high in this prebiotic fiber. Few of these foods are usually included in a diet for those who suffer from SIBO and IBS, as it is thought that resistant starch probably ferments prematurely before it reaches the large intestine due to the overgrowth of bacteria in the small intestine.

You may have already guessed it: I'm fascinated by fiber. Researchers from the American Gut Project – currently the world's largest study of the human microbiome – found that people who eat more than thirty different plants per week have optimal gut diversity and, consequently, better health. I use a lot of plant-based foods in my cooking and am always on the lookout for different varieties like red, yellow or purple carrots to ensure a varied diet. Not only do I love my veggies, but I am also a fan of the easily digestible red lentils and moong dhal (that's mung dhal without the green skin) because they can be used to make wonderful dishes like creamy soups or even sauces. If you soak moong dhal in water for a few hours, rinse it and puree it with some liquid – add some spices or herbs - you can even make pancakes out of it. Serve it with steamed vegetables like fennel, zucchini or squash and you have a light lunch or dinner.

## BUTYRATE

Many studies have shown that a high-fiber diet can improve brain function. This has been well demonstrated in children who followed such a diet, as their cognitive capabilities, memory, concentration, and ability to multitask, were better than in children who ate a low-fiber diet. The reason for this outcome may be the close relationship between a SCFA called butyrate and the brain. When the intestinal bacteria are fed with the right food, they form butyrate. Although it is primarily delivered to intestinal cells, some is bypassed via the portal vein and absorbed in the liver. Interestingly, an increase in the level of butyrate in the blood is observed mainly in people who eat a high-fiber diet.

Butyrate provides energy to the cells in the intestinal tissue. It is known for its ability to repair and improve the epithelial cells of the intestine, preventing increased permeability, that is, leaky gut. It has anti-inflammatory properties, which play an important role in cell reproduction and apoptosis. The latter is a regular, orderly cellular suicide that takes with it potentially dangerous cells such as cancer and virus-infected cells. Without the energy provided by butyrate, cells would be subject to self-destruction to a much greater extent. Butyrate may also relieve symptoms of ulcerative colitis, protect against colon cancer, improve motility and reduce visceral hypersensitivity. The latter condition manifests as severe pain in the internal organs and is a hallmark of IBS. Of course, there are other SCFAs such as acetate and propionate that contribute to our health, but the benefits of butyrate are particularly highlighted by researchers.

The name butyrate comes from the Greek word βουτυρος, which means butter. Butter is one of the valuable food sources for the formation of this molecule. Butter contains butyric acid in the form of triglycerides. Of course, butter is not the only source of butyrate. Other sources include breast milk and dairy products such as ghee, raw and cultured butter, Jersey milk, natural cheeses such as Emmental and Parmesan. There is even some butyrate in sauerkraut, vegetable oils and animal fats. To get the most benefit from animal foods, choose high-quality products from livestock that have been fed exclusively on pasture.

The highest butyric acid production comes from the bacteria in our gut. Their irrepressible urge to ferment dietary fiber is to our advantage. They love to nibble on resistant starch foods such as artichokes, asparagus, bananas, carrots, garlic, onions, beans, rice, and potatoes, and all whole grains, legumes, fruits, and vegetables. Unfortunately, many of the foods that promote butyrate production worsen symptoms of SIBO and IBS. To get around this problem, supplementation with butyrate could be a solution. Like Dr. Nigh says: "Anybody with digestive symptoms is going to benefit from butyrate".

# DAIRY

Mother's milk is the most important source of nutrients for all mammalian infants before they can digest any other food. After our mothers wean us, we usually consume the milk of animals such as cows, sheep, goats and occasionally buffalo, camels, reindeer, donkeys, horses or yak. The most popular is cow's milk and it accounts for 80% of the world's dairy supply. Milk consists of water, carbohydrates, fat, protein, vitamins, minerals, and enzymes. Not only does it have all nine essential amino acids that humans need, but it also has the most complex fatty acid composition of all edible fats.

The nutritional values of dairy products depends on the region and country where they are produced. The carbohydrate in milk is mainly lactose, the sugar molecules of which are a disaccharide consisting of glucose and galactose. Many people cannot tolerate lactose, and the food industry is meeting this demand with lactose-free products. Common symptoms of lactose intolerance are abdominal pain, bloating, fullness, and diarrhea. For some people, symptoms can be triggered by even a small amount of dairy; others are luckier as symptoms occur only after consuming large amounts. Lactose malabsorption can have various causes. For example, people with celiac disease, lactose cannot be processed because the enzyme lactase, which is responsible for breaking down lactose, is missing. For those with SIBO and IBS, the bacterial population in the small intestine likes to feed on this enzyme, making it unavailable to break down lactose.

The first time I realized I might have a serious problem with dairy was when I was out on a nice day with a group of friends. We were walking along the coast and stopped at a coffee bar where I had a large milkshake. On the way back, one of my friends noticed that I looked very bloated. The further we walked, the bigger my belly got until I looked like I was five months pregnant. Further experimentation with dairy confirmed my conclusion that it

> must have been the milkshake. How little did I know back then that this intolerance was probably related to celiac disease and gut imbalance.

Last but not least, lactose intolerance can be triggered by a parasite called *Giardia duodenalis* (*Giardia*). This aquatic parasite is common throughout the world and is transmitted via food or direct contact. Streams, wells, lakes, swimming pools, and municipal water supplies are the habitats of this microscopic organism. It usually disappears from the body within a few weeks, but gastrointestinal problems can last longer. Similar troublesome parasites include *Entamoeba coli* (*E. coli* for short and not to be confused with bacterium *Escherichia coli*) and *Dientamoeba fragilis*. The latter parasite lives in the gastrointestinal tract of humans, pigs, and gorillas. Symptoms are rare, but when they do occur, they may include loose stools, diarrhea, and abdominal pain. In children, infection is associated with loss of appetite, weight loss, nausea, fatigue, and failure to thrive. These parasites spread via fecal-oral ingestion, that is, consumption of contaminated food or water. Even if you have no signs of a parasitic infection, you can still be a host and pass it on. A stool test can clarify whether parasites are the cause of lactose intolerance. In most cases, this intolerance is temporary and disappears once the gut is healed.

There are two common tests to detect an intolerance to lactose. First, the lactose tolerance blood test that looks for glucose in blood; and second, the hydrogen breath test that requires a drink of lactose-containing solution. A third option, but less common, is a stool test that is usually performed on infants and young children. The result of this test shows whether the lactose has been properly broken down by the body.

To some extent, all dairy products contain the casein protein. Milk, cheese, yogurt, milk kefir, and ice cream have higher levels of this protein, while butter and cream contain only traces of it. Among the different types of casein, beta-casein is the second most abundant protein which has an excellent nutritional balance of amino acids. Beta-casein from cow's milk has several gene mutations, of which A1 and A2 are the most common. Each of these types has a unique amino acid composition, genetic variation, and different functions. Depending on the bovine species, one or the other type dominates and can promote intolerance to this type of milk. The A1 type significantly prolongs the transition time in the gastrointestinal tract, partly by reducing contractions. Casein can be responsible for stomach pain, digestive problems, joint pain, fatigue, and behavioral changes. In severe cases, it can cause vomiting, hives, and breathing difficulty. To determine if you have a problem with this protein, you can perform a food specific immunoglobulin IgE skin prick test or a blood test to check for antibodies. Some laboratories offer a cross-reactive gliadin foods test, which examines alpha and beta-casein at the same time. Sometimes there is no indication of casein intolerance in the test results, but symptoms still occur. In this case, it may be helpful to follow an elimination diet, avoiding dairy products for at least one month. After this period, you can add a small amount of dairy that contains casein back into your diet. If the symptoms worsen again, you'll know what is causing it.

In addition to casein protein, dairy products contain whey protein, which seems to be less of a concern because it is absorbed quickly. Many athletes take whey protein shakes to recover better from workouts and to build muscle. Other people take it to lose weight, because it can curb appetite and stimulate metabolism. Researchers found that taking a whey supplement increased the synthesis of the antioxidant glutathione, and improved muscle strength in patients with Parkinson's disease. The whey family consists mainly of beta-lactoglobulin, alpha-lactalbumin, lactoferrin, immunoglobulins, serum albumin, and enzymes. It is also a transporter of nutrients, has anti-inflammatory effects, and helps the body fight infection. On the negative side, it can cause fatigue, headaches, loss of appetite, thirst, and like casein, increase intestinal discomfort such as bloating and cramps. A whey protein powder is generally safe if you do not have an allergy or intolerance to dairy products. But beware – many of these products contain corn, soy, or even artificial ingredients that can aggravate symptoms. Special care should also be taken during pregnancy or breastfeeding, as it is not yet known whether whey protein powder is safe for infants. If you want to know if a milk protein is causing you problems, you can do an allergy blood test that looks for IgE antibodies or specific tests that search for the alpha-lactalbumin, beta-lactoglobulin and the casein protein.

Dairy is such a tricky ingredient – on the one hand, it has many benefits, especially when it comes from a grass-fed animal as then it has particularly high anti-inflammatory and healing properties. It provides essential fat-soluble vitamins, and protects the body from oxidative stress. Fermented dairy products are also excellent probiotics. On the other hand, dairy can lead to all sorts of problems such as inflammation and gut dysbiosis. It can alter hormone levels, which can contribute to a higher risk of developing breast, colon, and prostate cancer. Dairy products can increase mucus production in the intestine that impacts the mucosa and may lead to poor absorption of nutrients. In some cases, the body may even develop antibodies to dairy and treat the milk protein like gluten. Weighing all the pros and cons of dairy, it is important that no food should be excluded from the diet unless it is absolutely necessary and the exclusion is by no means due to a fad.

If you can't tolerate dairy products like milk, you can try low-lactose foods, such as aged cheeses like Swiss, cheddar, and parmesan, a 24-hour fermented homemade yogurt, or commercially produced lactose-free dairy products. If you want to avoid dairy altogether, you can turn to vegan products and non-dairy milks such as almond, coconut, soy and oat milk.

Coconut products, including drinks, juices, milk, cream, and powder, have become very popular and are often used as dairy alternatives. Although they may give the impression that they are "dairy-free," caution is advised for people with a true dairy allergy or intolerance. In recent years, the Australian government has recalled several products from countries such as China, Taiwan, Malaysia, Thailand, and Vietnam because they did not contain the required allergy warning despite containing dairy. People have suffered severe allergic reactions or died after drinking what they believed was "dairy-free" coconut milk. If you are unsure about a product, check with the importer or manufacturer.

Cow's milk is not the only way to enjoy the nutritional properties of milk. Camel milk, for example, has been used for medical purposes for centuries in the Middle Eastern, Asian, and African cultures. It can be a nutritious alternative for people who react strongly to cow, sheep, or goat milk. If you are lucky enough to live in Australia, Saudi Arabia, or any other country where there are camels, you can get fresh, frozen, and powdered milk. The chemical composition of camel's milk is similar to that of human breast milk. However, it is not a substitute for infants, because they still need the real thing – breast milk or a proper infant formula. Some promising studies show that older children with milk allergies are able to tolerate camel's milk well. This milk contains very little lactose compared to cow's milk. It has a little sugar and cholesterol, but at the same time it is rich in minerals such as sodium, potassium, iron, copper, zinc, magnesium, and vitamin C. In fermented form, it is said to be a good remedy for diarrhea. Although it contains some caseins and whey, it does not seem to trigger typical immune reactions. Camel milk has a distinctive taste – slightly salty, but refreshing.

Unfortunately, I haven't had a chance to try fresh camel milk yet, but the other day I bought a marinated feta cheese made from camel milk. It was delicious and tasted like the goat milk feta from my local farmer's market. This taste and the fact that camel milk is a natural prebiotic, rich in nutrients, minerals and vitamins encouraged me to order a powder from a camel farm in Queensland, Australia. It might be a nice change of pace, since I'm a little tired of dairy substitutes such as coconut milk and almond milk – oat milk isn't necessarily safe for celiac disease as I explained in the previous chapter – and both hemp and soy milk don't really appeal to me.

Lait de jument – or, in English, mare's milk – could be another option for people with an intolerance to cow's milk. Although it contains casein and a high percentage of lactose, it requires only half the digestion time compared to cow's milk because its chemical structure is similar to human milk. Mare's milk is low in fat and cholesterol, and contains vitamins and minerals including vitamins A, B, C and E, potassium, iron, calcium, and magnesium. It has a slightly sweet, grassy, and nutty taste. I wasn't convinced after trying a powdered version from France that my friend had enthusiastically told me about. Perhaps I would have had a different experience drinking fresh milk instead of the powdered version. Nonetheless, my personal preferences shouldn't stop you from trying it for yourself. Mare's milk is available in some European countries but also in Russia and Mongolia. In the traditional medicine of these two countries, it is used to treat diseases of the cardiovascular system, beriberi, anemia, allergies, and gastrointestinal diseases such as Crohn's disease, ulcerative colitis, hepatitis, and chronic gastric ulcers. It is used as a laxative, fermented to produce a low-alcohol beverage, and incorporated in a variety of cosmetics to treat skin problems, including atopic dermatitis. Due to its enzymes, including lactoferrin and lysozyme, it even stimulates and strengthens the immune system.

## GHEE

Ghee has been around for thousands of years and is used extensively in Ayurvedic medicine and Indian cuisine. It is made from butter that has been clarified by removing the solid components of the milk. Although it is made from milk, it may be suitable for some people with dairy intolerance as the manufacturing process reduces the substances that usually cause problems. It is solid when chilled and liquid when warm or heated. Ghee is very high in saturated fat and is a popular cooking fat in many countries as it has an excellent shelf life and a high smoking point of 482°F (250°C). One tablespoon of this fat has around 123 kcal

(515 KJ). It offers macronutrients like calcium, vitamins A, E and K, and beta carotene.

Not all researchers agree on whether ghee is beneficial or not. One concern is that the high saturated fat content increases the risk of cardiovascular disease. Other studies refute this fear and say that ghee consumption led to lower cholesterol, triglyceride, and phospholipid levels. Ghee, enjoyed in moderation, could be a healthy choice as it contains SCFAs, which support digestion, cell membrane growth and reduces inflammation. It's all a matter of dietary balance and how ghee is used in food preparation. Frying and sautéing with it can be less beneficial than using it as a spread on bread or as a medicine with some herbs. The flavor of ghee depends greatly on the brand and source of ingredients. There are a variety of commercial ghee products that can range from nutty buttery to oily and slightly stale. If you have never tried it, I would recommend buying an organic and "grass-fed" product, as it has a more pleasant taste and contains higher amounts of butyrate and other nutrients. Keep in mind that casein content can vary greatly from brand to brand, from high to nonexistent. If you want to be absolutely certain, contact the manufacturer for more information. Even with homemade ghee, you can't be sure how much casein is still present. Depending on your sensitivity to lactose and casein, it may not be safe for you.

# CONCEPT SUMMARY

» All humans need carbohydrates, proteins, and fats to survive. These essential macronutrients have specific molecular structures and functions. Carbohydrates consist of simple sugar, proteins consist of amino acids, and fats consist of fatty acids. Some people have difficulty tolerating these molecules.

» FODMAPs are sugar molecules found in carbohydrates. People with IBS and SIBO often have difficulty processing these sugars, which is why they experience bothersome symptoms.

» Every part of our physical body needs amino acids, and since amino acids can't be stored, they must be supplied daily from food. There are twenty different amino acids, but only nine of them are called "essential" because they cannot be synthesized by the body. Certain proteins can cause allergic reactions or intolerances in some people.

» Fatty acids are essential for many bodily functions including organs, tissues, and hormone production. Not all fats are equally healthy, and some need to be consumed with more caution. This is especially true for saturated fats.

» Dietary fiber is the ultimate for health. For people with SIBO and IBS, some varieties can cause problems. Regardless of your health condition, you should not lose sight of integrating fiber into your diet.

» Butyrate is the main energy supplier to maintain and renew intestinal cells. This SCFA is produced in larger quantities during the metabolism of dietary fiber by bacteria in the large intestine. A supplement can be useful if certain foods are not well tolerated.

» Milk is a valuable food that contains all nine essential amino acids and is a rich source of antibodies. On the other hand, it is one of the most difficult ingredients for the body to process. One or all of its components, such as lactose, casein, and whey, can be the cause of numerous symptoms.

# GLUTEN

Since gluten is such a hot topic, I will go into more detail to give you a deeper insight. There is no doubt that gluten causes problems for some people who can't tolerate it or suffer from celiac disease. Still, not every intestinal reaction means gluten is the culprit. It is possible that some symptoms are caused by carbohydrates. So, before you eliminate an entire food group that contains gluten from your diet, you should gather more information and possibly get tested for celiac disease.

## WHAT IS GLUTEN?

When a plant attempts to reproduce, it releases its offspring with a care package – the seed. It contains a variety of substances such as starch, oils, fiber, vitamins, minerals, and proteins that nourish the embryonic plant during the germination period. To ensure successful growth and protection, the germ has additional tools that are stored in the seed. One of these is the endosperm, which surrounds the offspring and provides nutrients in the form of starch. It also contains prolamin, which is found mainly in plants such as grains. Each seed family has a specific composition of proteins in its prolamin container that can react upon contact with another element to form a new substance. For example, when the wheat proteins gliadin and glutenin are mixed with water, gluten is formed. Gluten itself has little nutritional value, but bakers love it because it gives dough an elastic consistency and helps the bread retain its shape during rising and baking. The downside side of gluten is that it can be difficult to digest because it is insoluble in water and has a glue-like consistency. This fact seems to be one of the main causes of many undesirable symptoms. Gluten-forming proteins are also present in many other grains such as barley, rye, spelt, wheat, ferro, triticale, semolina, and Khorasan wheat, also known as kamut in some regions.

However, don't confuse gluten with the glutinous protein in rice and corn that makes them sticky when cooked.

The gliadin protein can affect zonulin – remember the bouncer in the intestinal wall that decides what can or cannot enter the bloodstream? When bribed, it loosens the cells of the digestive wall and releases unwanted antigens into circulation, causing inflammation and leaky gut. The body is normally able to digest proteins easily, but gluten protein is quite resistant to digestion in the stomach and small intestines. It is not always completely broken down and instead ends up as peptides, which are protein particles made up of smaller amino acid chains with unique binding properties. In principle, there are many different types of peptides that have a wide range of physical functions. For example, they can control our body's responses to food and physical activity and influence how neurotransmitters and hormones work. Normally, any undigested constituents of gluten pass through the digestive tract and are excreted without signs of intolerance, but there are exceptions.

## CELIAC DISEASE

Celiac disease is also known as coeliac sprue, non-tropical sprue, idiopathic sprue, idiopathic steatorrhea and gluten-sensitive enteropathy. It is an autoimmune disorder that occurs in genetically predisposed individuals and is manifested by gluten intolerance. Affected people may develop symptoms such as diarrhea, constipation, nausea, vomiting, flatulence, bloating, abdominal pain, fatigue, weight loss or gain, bone and joint aches, psoriasis, skin rashes, frequent bruising, leaky gut and malabsorption. The latter is often associated with deficiency in iron, vitamin B12, folic acid and calcium since the damaged villi can no longer adequately absorb these nutrients. Some people experience sensory symptoms such as pain, tingling and numbness in the feet and fingertips, or even facial pain. Still others have no symptoms at all. Associated diseases are type 1 diabetes, Down's syndrome, Turner

syndrome, thyroid conditions, hepatitis, infertility, dermatitis herpeti-
formis, liver disease, chronic pancreatitis, gluten ataxia, SIBO and IBS.
The more indirect consequences of this disease are lactose intolerance,
anemia, recurrent mouth ulcers, early onset of osteopenia and osteoporosis, altered mental alertness and irritability. Children can experience
poor growth and failure to thrive or delayed puberty.

In celiac disease, gluten peptides bind to antigen cells, which then
enter the intestinal mucosa. There they interact with T cells - which
are part of the immune system army - and trigger an inflammatory
response. The villi of a celiac disease patient are damaged and may be
reduced to the point where they are just a flat surface; this condition
is called villous atrophy. Three main factors favor the development of
celiac disease: first, a genetic predisposition with the antigens HLA-
DQ2 and HLA-DQ8; second, exposure to gluten-containing food, and
third, increased permeability of the intestinal mucosal barrier - leaky
gut. The likelihood of developing this disease increases if celiac disease
runs in your family and you are of Caucasian descent. The HLA antigens
are quite common and do not alone indicate an increased risk. Celiac
disease can occur at any age if the above conditions are met.

Before a diagnosis of celiac disease can be made, it is essential to
consume gluten regularly for several weeks prior to testing, otherwise
the result can be inaccurate or difficult to interpret. Currently, the first
step in diagnosis is a blood test, usually based on ELISA, which may
include anti-gliadin, anti-endomysial, anti-transglutaminase, or deami-
dated gluten peptide antibodies. Even if the blood test is positive, there
is still a possibility that the individual does not have celiac disease. The
next step is to verify the result through a gastroscopy (or endoscopy),
in which a small, thin, flexible tube with a light and camera is inserted
through the mouth to view the stomach, esophagus, and first part of the
small intestine. The gastroenterologist will conduct a biopsy to assess the
degree of damage to the villi and rule out other diseases such as Crohn's
disease. In some cases, especially in young children, gastrointestinal

endoscopy may not be necessary, but this must be discussed with the pediatric gastroenterologist. The pathologist analyzes the biopsy using specific criteria based on the Marsh classification system that was developed by M. N. Marsh in 1992 and later modified by G. Oberhuber and his colleagues in 1999. The current Marsh-Oberhuber classification ranges from Marsh I to Marsh IV, with Marsh III divided into IIIa, IIIb and IIIc. Normally, people with celiac disease fall into the Marsh III category but there are more and more people who test negative for this disease but have Marsh I and II, possibly due to the sensitivity of the tests available today. A milder degree of enteropathy does not equate to a mild disease. Dr. Bulsiewicz has observed that people with Marsh I and II respond well to a gluten-free diet. He recommends that if celiac disease is suspected, it is essential to test for genetic predisposition (antigens) and perform an endoscopy as the blood test cannot detect low grades of enteropathy.

I learned firsthand what Dr. Bulsiewicz observed. Several years before I was diagnosed with celiac disease, the blood test came back negative, which made me feel like I was on the safe side. However, I still had many of the symptoms associated with the disease. Over the next few years, my health continued to go downhill until an endoscopy brought more clarity. At this point, my villi had become quite flat, and I was suffering from severe nutrient deficiencies. My doctor provided me with vitamin and iron shots to counteract this condition, and I switched to a gluten-free diet. But that wasn't the end of my health journey, as the side effects of this disease such as osteopenia, lactose intolerance, IBS and SIBO still keep me on my toes.

A diagnosis of celiac disease means a lifelong avoidance of gluten. Cheating is not allowed. Even if you feel much better after following a gluten-free diet, don't be tempted to eat gluten ever again. It can trigger a severe reaction and further damage to the small intestine, which can potentially be life-threatening in some circumstances. There are cases in which celiac disease patients do not get well after switching to a gluten-free diet. The reason for this may be cross-reactive foods, that is, foods that are contaminated with gluten. Hence, one should pay special attention to foods such as yeast, instant coffee, chocolate, corn, oats, millet, rice, and quinoa. The latter food is a little tricky, as some varieties can trigger an immune reaction, while others are well tolerated in small quantities. The casein protein from dairy can also be a confounding factor, as it can cause an inflammatory response similar to a gluten response. If symptoms do not improve despite a strict gluten-free diet and avoidance of the foods listed above, dysbiosis, IBS and SIBO may also be present. It is common for celiac patients to have an overgrowth of various bacteria, such as *Bacteriodes*, *Proteobacteria*, *Prevotella*, *E. coli*, *Clostridium*, as well as a decrease in *Bifidobacterium* and *Firmicutes* bacteria. Unhealthy levels of *Streptococcaceae* bacteria can also be found, either too high or too low concentrations. Researchers found that patients who continued a strict gluten-free diet and were treated with antibiotics suitable for SIBO had no further symptoms.

## NON-CELIAC GLUTEN SENSITIVITY

Scientists are still in the dark about why some people who don't have celiac disease still develop similar symptoms when they eat gluten, albeit often with more headaches, foggy brain, depression, and anxiety. These people feel much better once they stop eating gluten. However, the clinical picture differs from that of a person with celiac disease, as there is no evidence of villi atrophy or celiac-specific antibodies; instead, elevated level of anti-gliadin IgG and white blood cells (lymphocytes) may be present.

While many people switch to a gluten-free diet after self-diagnosis, not all are actually gluten sensitive or intolerant. Some may have a wheat allergy, which can manifest as asthma and rhinitis - as seen in baker's asthma - or may develop skin and gastrointestinal tract issues. If it is a true allergy, symptoms may appear within a few hours after eating products containing gluten or inhaling these flours. In severe cases anaphylaxis can occur. Some people may react to the various components of the grain, including the carbohydrate oligos. They can trigger water retention in the intestines and increased gas production – both of which lead to a prominent upper abdomen. As mentioned earlier, oligos belong to the FODMAP group and are found in wheat, garlic, onion, artichokes, dried apricots, cashews, pistachio, soy, beans, lentils, and chickpeas. Other causes of adverse reactions may be chemicals in the grain that are part of the plant's defense strategy. They can affect digestive enzymes, resulting in inadequately digested food that weakens the immune system. Perhaps the problem may be anti-nutrients such as lectin, phytates, tannins, and oxalates, which bind important micronutrients and prevent them from being absorbed by the body. Although these plant components are usually well tolerated, some people experience adverse effects. To reduce the level of anti-nutrient substances in foods, they can be prepared accordingly. For example, plant foods that contain lectins such as grains and legumes are less aggravating when soaked and thoroughly cooked, fermented, or sprouted. With one exemption: sprouted (raw) red kidney beans are poisonous due to their high lectin content.

Don't underestimate how difficult it is to distinguish between diseases with similar symptoms. It is not an easy task for your doctor or healthcare provider to make the correct diagnosis. If you have more than one disorder, it becomes even more complicated. For example, celiac disease, lactose intolerance and SIBO mimics IBS symptoms, while giardiasis mimics celiac disease. A person with IBS may feel better after avoiding gluten, as may someone with non-celiac gluten sensitivity (NCGS), or perhaps not. A person with celiac disease may give up eating gluten but still experience bloating. Someone with SIBO may be on a low-FODMAP diet and avoid gluten but still react to many other foods, and so forth. The first approach is not to go on a gluten-free diet until you have seen a doctor. If you have been off gluten for a while, it can be difficult to rule out celiac disease. If you have already changed your diet, you may need to do a gluten challenge for up to eight weeks before you can be tested for this disease.

Gluten-free diets are currently in vogue. A wide range of products is offered in stores but they are not always the best choice, even for those who must eat gluten-free for medical reasons. Not only are these products expensive, but they are also usually highly processed, and therefore have low nutritional value and too little fiber. The lack of nutrients and minerals such as vitamin D, B12, folic acid, iron, zinc, magnesium, and calcium in these products is a concern, especially for women who are pregnant or want to become so. Folic acid, also known as vitamin B9, is essential for a healthy baby. Another worry is that a gluten-free diet carries a higher risk of arsenic and mercury exposure. American researchers analyzed data from over seven thousand people, about 1.2% of whom reported being on a gluten-free diet. This group had twice as much arsenic in their urine and about 70% more mercury in their blood. The cause is thought to be rice flour, which is often used as a substitute for gluten-containing grains and is known to be a potent carrier of these toxic chemicals. The other assumption is that a gluten-free diet often does not contain enough fiber to help to transport these chemicals out of the body. A member of this research group, Maria Argos, says more research needs to be done to determine whether a gluten-free diet poses a health risk. She points out that in the United States there are no regulations for detecting metals in food, while in Europe, at least exposure to arsenic is regulated.

A gluten-free diet is not a lifestyle choice or a means to lose weight. Trying to use it as a weight-loss tool could be counterproductive, because research shows that people on a gluten-free diet are more likely to gain weight as they generally eat more calories and less dietary fiber. Most gluten-free products such as breads, muffins and cookies have a high glycemic index (GI), which indicates how quickly food is broken down into glucose sugars and absorbed by the body. If the GI is high and the food is broken down too quickly, we soon get hungry again and want more. On the other hand, if the GI is low, metabolism takes longer and blood sugar level remains stable, keeping us satisfied for longer.

A strict gluten-free diet is not easy to maintain, as many everyday products contain hidden gluten, such as soy sauce, chocolate, take-away food, flavor enhancers, dietary supplements, medications, toothpaste, and herbs. Reading labels is crucial, and when eating out, be sure to check all the ingredients that make up the meal. Even if everything seems fine, you can never be one hundred percent sure that no gluten has been smuggled in through contamination. Try to prepare your own meals with plenty of fresh ingredients as often as possible. Don't be tempted by the "gluten-free" aisle at the supermarket to meet your needs. Plan your meals in advance and pack food in a travel cooler when you're on the road. Invite friends over for dinner that you've prepared or give them clear instructions on how and what to cook when they cook for you.

> When I was diagnosed with celiac disease, I switched to a gluten-free diet and had to make some small changes in my kitchen. It was important to avoid all sources of contamination, which meant a new cutting board and toaster came into our household. My relatives and friends are supportive and do their best to offer me alternatives when I am invited to dinner or a party. It's so nice that some even bake cakes especially for me. Unfortunately, I still have to be vigilant, like when a relative proudly presented her gluten-free homemade cake and said that she only used a small amount of wheat flour to dust the cake pan. I wasn't sure who was more disappointed.

## A WORD ON OATS

Oat is a highly nutritious, naturally gluten-free grain. It contains proteins, soluble (beta-glucan) and insoluble fiber, vitamins, especially B-complex, antioxidants and iron. The main protein is avenalin, which is similar to the proteins of legumes. The other, but less abundant protein avenin is related to wheat gluten. Generally, its protein is smaller than that of wheat and can form a bond with sulfur. When oats are consumed regularly, they increase the production of butyrate and positively alter the microbiome. They are also beneficial for inflammatory bowel diseases such as ulcerative colitis, colorectal adenomas, and cancer. But oats aren't just oats, as there are many varieties and origins of this grain. Some varieties trigger immune reactions, while others do not. This is due to the different amino acid sequence of the respective oat protein.

People with celiac disease must be careful when eating oats because, like gluten, it can cause intestinal inflammation and villi atrophy. This is due to cross-contamination with wheat, barley, and rye as these grains grow side by side in the fields and are often processed in the same facilities. Celiac Australia recommends having an endoscopy before adding oats to your diet and repeating this screening three months later to determine if oats are safe for you. In my eyes, that's a lot of effort for a few breakfast oats. Buying certified gluten-free oats may be the easier way to go. Manufacturers of gluten-free oats commonly use mechanical and/or optical sorting technologies that separate the oats from the gluten-containing grains at all stages of production. The products are further tested to ensure that manufacturers deliver what they promise. Gluten-free oats are available in the United States and Europe and are imported to Australia and New Zealand. Due to the food laws in the latter two countries, a product cannot be labeled "gluten-free" until it contains less than 3 ppm (parts per million) or 3mg/kg of gluten. This calculation does not include ingredients such as glucose syrup, dextrose, and caramel color, which are often found in gluten-free products but are derived from gluten-containing grains. In comparison, the European Union, the United Kingdom, and the United States allow gluten-free products to be labeled up to 20 ppm; this value includes all added ingredients used. People with celiac disease are advised not to eat products containing more than 20ppm of gluten. This corresponds to an Australian oat product that is labeled as "wheat-free". In case you are less restricted with gluten than a person with celiac disease, you can choose a low-gluten product with 100 ppm or less. If you experience discomfort with oats, it may not be due to gluten, but an increase in dietary fiber, its FODMAPs, or a reaction to the oat protein itself. Before adding oats to your diet you may like to discuss this topic with your doctor or nutritionist, as monitoring of antibody levels may be required.

# DIETS

With both IBS and SIBO, following a specific diet is an integral part of the treatment. The basic principle of these diets is to eliminate or reduce certain food groups to provide immediate symptom relief, control bacteria, and ensure adequate nutrition. However, they do not cure these diseases and should not be used as a permanent solution as they lack nutritional diversity. Diversity is the key to a healthy microbiome, which can easily be compared to that of a rainforest. Its inhabitants are a collection of microbes, bacteria, archaea, viruses, and even symbiotic parasites, all forming a healthy community. When this ecosystem is disturbed, parts are cleared or become stunted, allowing some microorganisms to take control. This is where the trouble begins. The aim is to bring this system back into a healthy balance, which is particularly supported by a diverse diet. A healthy balance is not supported if your diet is one-sided and mainly dominated by certain ingredients, for example potato, corn, rice, and wheat. Toast in the morning, pasta for lunch, cookies in the afternoon and pizza for dinner could be an example of a typical wheat day. With this type of diet, it is difficult for the body to compensate for the lack of other important nutrients. A characteristic of all mono diets is that the diversity in the microbiome dwindles.

It is commonly believed that we eat a much more diverse diet than nanna and pop did in the good old days when they only ate the produce from their garden. It seems logical to us that food diversity should have increased, since we now have access to foods from all over the world. Scientists have proved us wrong. Australian researchers led by Michael Bird of the James Cook University in Cairns analyzed 14,000 tissue samples from past and present humans. They concluded that a hundred years ago - before the invention of artificial fertilizers, industrialized agriculture and livestock - people had a much greater variety of plant and animal foods than we have today. This dietary diversity was most evident among self-supporting and small communities. With the advent of supermarkets and modern agriculture, there are now fewer plant and animal species than ever before. These researchers note that the modern diet is "in stark contrast" to past eating practices, where we sourced our food from our immediate environment. After all, as omnivores, we were able to feed on the entire terrestrial and marine ecosystem of the planet. With today's mono agriculture and globalization, our food palette has shrunk dramatically by two-thirds, compared to the past.

Every day anew we decide what to eat to nourish ourselves. Although farmers' markets, greengrocers and supermarkets offer many fresh products, we often ignore them because we succumb to the temptation of convenience. We pack unhealthy and processed favorites into our shopping carts because they promise a quick meal after a long day. Day after day, it's the same game all over the world. I can understand why, but we shouldn't be surprised that with a constant bombardment of nutrient-poor foods our bodies have trouble staying healthy. Yet, we can do something about it by changing our diet and eating more dietary fiber, because it supports the growth of health-promoting microorganisms and reduces undesirable ones. It's like joining a rainforest regeneration group: weed, replant, nurture. Change doesn't come overnight, but if we put in the effort, we'll soon see positive results.

The microbiome is strongly influenced by what we eat. Carbohydrates and sugar are the preferred foods on which certain types of bacteria thrive especially well. For this reason, IBS and SIBO diets exclude these foods to some degree to help to reduce bloating and inflammation. The most common diet for IBS is the low-FODMAP diet, which can also be used for SIBO. However, there are also other diets for SIBO. Currently, the most popular ones are the SIBO Specific Food Guide and the SIBO Bi-Phasic Diet, but these are not the only diets you can consider. Below you can find a brief description of these and some alternative diets.

Just a word of caution. People who are severely underweight must consult a doctor before starting any of these restricted diets to rule out serious diseases such as cancer or inflammation. After that, it is advisable to consult a nutritionist to ensure that enough calories are consumed.

## SPECIFIC CARBOHYDRATE DIET

Today's dietary approach to IBS and SIBO began in 1924, when New York pediatrician Dr. Sidney V. Haas was desperate to find a cure for what is now known as celiac disease. He experimented with banana flour and plantain meal and achieved excellent results for his diarrhea patients. For this reason, the diet earned the nickname "banana diet". Dr. Haas concluded that eliminating carbohydrates, refined sugars, gluten and starches not only dramatically improved his patients' symptoms, but also enabled them to heal completely without having any relapses. For nutritional reasons, he later reintroduced specific carbohydrates into the diet. In 1951, he and his son, Dr. Merrill P. Haas, wrote the medical textbook *Management of Celiac Disease*. Until his death, Dr. Sidney Haas believed that carbohydrates were the cause of celiac disease, although Dutch pediatrician W.K. Dick proved in the 1950s that the wheat protein and not starch was the culprit.

The biochemist and cell biologist Elaine Gottschall was a huge fan of Dr. Haas. Her daughter Judy suffered from ulcerative colitis at an early age and was one of Dr. Haas' patients. Doctors gave Ms. Gottschall no hope other than to agree to surgery to remove her daughter's colon and attach an external bag to collect her excretions. Dr. Haas was the first to ask her what her daughter was eating. Within two years of following his diet, Judy was symptom free. Later, Ms. Gottschall used her profession to further develop this diet. She was a pioneer of classifying carbohydrates according to their molecular structure and digestibility. In her view, certain carbohydrates feed harmful intestinal bacteria that can cause an overgrowth and lead to inflammation of the intestinal mucosa. She suspected that people with gastrointestinal disorders have damaged or missing enzymes that cannot break down simple carbohydrates such as sugars and starches. To regain balance in the gastrointestinal system she recommends starving unwanted bacteria by eliminating specific carbohydrates. She advocates this diet for treating Crohn's disease, ulcerative colitis, diverticulitis, cystic fibrosis, chronic diarrhea, and autism. Her book, *Breaking the Vicious Cycle. Intestinal Health Through Diet* is still a standard work for many today. Ms. Gottschall's official website, named after the book, provides information and an overview of foods that may help heal the gut.

The SCD is currently gaining attention in the scientific world due to a greater interest in conducting clinical research on nutritional therapies and finding a treatment for irritable bowel disease. An observational study showed that a patient with ulcerative colitis and primary sclerosing cholangitis achieved positive results after using the SCD, although some dominant bacterial species in the patient's microbiome were not reduced. David Suskind, clinician and a pediatric gastroenterologist at Seattle Children's Hospital, confirms this positive outcome as he uses the SCD successfully for his Crohn's and ulcerative colitis patients.

My experience with SCD goes back several years. At the time, I was frustrated because I wasn't getting enough help from my doctor to relieve my symptoms of rosacea, bloating and constipation. While looking for help, I came across the website Wright/Reasoner SCD Lifestyle (now Healthy Gut) and followed their version of the SCD. This diet is not for the faint-hearted. The first month was the most challenging for me, but after that it got easier. After three months, I was able to eat exactly ten different foods plus meat. I have to say I felt fantastic, and my stomach has never been so flat. Unfortunately, after reintroducing more foods, my symptoms slowly and steadily returned. My doctor recommended that I expand my diet to include more nutrients and suggested a food intolerance test. Oddly enough, all the foods I ate during SCD showed elevated IgG levels. It was obvious to my doctor that I also must have leaky gut. In hindsight, I would not do this type of diet again unless absolutely necessary. It was too strict, and I felt quite socially isolated and stressed.

## LOW-FODMAP DIET

FODMAPs are widespread in our diet. People who have problems with these substances often develop symptoms such as water and gas formation in the intestines, which in turn causes bloating, discomfort and pain in the abdomen. To alleviate symptoms, FODMAP-containing foods should be avoided or greatly reduced.

The low-FODMAP diet has a worldwide reputation for being effective in the treatment of IBS. About 50-80% of patients with IBS respond well to this diet, especially if they have a mild form of the disease or if they suffer predominantly from diarrhea; it seems less effective for constipation. Researchers at Monash University point out that it is not an elimination diet, even though it restricts certain food groups. The LDF is not meant to be followed indefinitely, as long-term avoidance of these food groups can lead to a loss of diversity in the microbiome. It is best to consult a nutritionist to guide you through the entire FODMAP program to avoid nutrient deficiencies. This program consists of three phases. During the first two to six weeks, the diet must be strictly adhered to. This is followed by a reintroduction of the respective food groups for up to six to eight weeks. Then, the diet is adapted to individual needs. Since food intolerances can change over time, it is advisable to regularly check whether the relevant foods are still tolerated. Many foods that contain FODMAPs have prebiotic substances such as butyrate. When these foods are avoided, the development of beneficial bacteria is inhibited. With this in mind, and due to lack of research on the long-term effects of this diet, it is not yet clear how safe LDF is over a long period of time. The question seems to be how to find the right balance between symptoms and an adequate nutritional intake. If you want to try this diet, you can buy a mobile app for iOS and Android from the Monash University. It takes the guesswork out of which foods belong to which food group. You can also buy a small booklet or check out their blog for more information. Fortunately, FODMAPs are water soluble so they cannot dissolve in oil. This knowledge works to your advantage, as you can use it to make a garlic-infused oil that can add flavor to your meals. Take a small pan and fry one or more cloves of garlic with a little oil, discard the cloves, and use the infused oil for your dish. Don't be tempted to chop or puree the garlic cloves as it will be much harder to remove all solids from the oil. Any contact with garlic solids and the watery contents of meat or vegetables would result in fructans leaching out, making the dish high in FODMAPs. You can also buy garlic-infused, low-FODMAP oils online and in stores.

## SIBO SPECIFIC FOOD GUIDE

While in medical school, Dr. Siebecker was desperate for a solution to her chronic gastrointestinal complaints and discovered Elaine Gottschall's book. After implementing this dietary approach with great results, she wanted to gain a deeper understanding of it. In her research, she discovered that there was a link between Gottschall's description of gastrointestinal symptoms, and the term "Small Intestinal Bacterial Overgrowth" used by gastroenterologists in their work in the late 1990s. With this insight, she brought science and diet together. Since then, she has dedicated herself to finding a cure for SIBO and helps people to overcome this disease. She developed the SIBO Specific Food Guide, which is a combination of the SCD diet and the low-FODMAP diet. The idea behind this diet is to starve bacteria by avoiding particular carbohydrates. Dr. Siebecker accomplishes this by dividing foods into "legal" and "illegal" foods. The latter category includes foods containing resistant starch and soluble fiber as well as prebiotics, any form of sugars – except for honey - processed meats like bacon, and many dairy products including kefir. Not to forget spices such as onion, garlic, balsamic vinegar, soy sauce and tamari, cocoa powder, and chocolate – even the unsweetened version –asafetida, and chicory. Of course, in this diet are many foods that can be eaten in moderation or are "legal".

Visit her website for a downloadable PDF of the SIBO Specific Food Guide. It is hidden under the heading "Treatment", and then "Diet". A free mobile app for iOS is found under "Resources".

## THE GUT AND PSYCHOLOGY SYNDROME DIET

Dr. Natasha Campbell-McBride, a Russian-trained medical doctor living in England with a postgraduate degree in neurology and human nutrition, is another person who was inspired by Elaine Gottschall's SCD. She was looking for a cure to help her son, who was diagnosed with autism in his early years. Frustrated that the medical world had little to offer them, she decided to try the SCD. Her son responded so well to this diet that in 1998 she decided to open a health clinic to help others with similar problems. However, her modified version of the SCD is far more restricted than the original diet. She calls it the "Gut and Psychology Syndrome Diet", or "GAPS" for short. Dr. Campbell-McBride believes that a dysfunctional gut-brain axis causes many neurological and psychiatric conditions. In 2004, she published her first book *Gut and Psychology Syndrome: Natural Treatment for Autism, Dyspraxia, A.D.D., Dyslexia, A.D.H.D., Depression, Schizophrenia*. Other books followed. The GAPS protocol is a multi-year treatment that focuses on detoxifying the body and cleaning the gastrointestinal tract to improve brain function. Her diet is divided into different stages: the preparation phase, introduction/detox phase, and the main treatment. It can take up to two years or more to reintroduce new foods. The GAPS diet gained popularity with the claim that it can help with various minor and serious diseases, but to date scientific evidence is lacking.

## CEDARS-SINAI DIET

Dr. Pimental was one of the first scientists to suggest that bacteria play a significant role in the development of IBS. In 2008, he published the book *A New IBS Solution. Bacteria–The Missing Link in Treating Irritable*

*Bowel Syndrome* and laid the foundation for further research into SIBO and IBS. His dietary approach, the Cedars-Sinai diet (C-SD), is used to prevent a relapse of SIBO and its cousin IBS after a successful treatment. The focus of this diet is on foods that are easy to digest and leave little food for bacteria to feast on. Dr. Pimental says eating simple and easily digestible carbohydrates like rice, potatoes, sweet potatoes, and pasta is acceptable, but they should not be reheated because then they become resistant starch. All types of white bread and sourdough bread are allowed, but not the whole grain or multigrain varieties. Dark chocolate and nuts seem to be okay, as well as oils, since bacteria can't digest them. Most fresh fruits are allowed, however, banana, apples and pears can slow motility and should be consumed only in small quantities. Compared to other SIBO and IBS elimination diets, C-SD allows onions and garlic – actually, anything that grows under the ground. The approach of the C-SD is to minimize restriction to prevent social isolation and therefore mental stress.

The C-SD avoids all insoluble carbohydrates, dairy products, and most sweeteners. Dr. Pimental says that sucrose (white sugar) and glucose are easy for humans to digest, while fructose (fruit sugar) and lactose (milk sugar) are harder to process. The worst offenders that fall under the "not absorbable" category are sucralose (splendaTM), sorbitol (sugar-free chewing gums), xylitol, lactulose, lactitol, and many other synthetically produced sugars. To limit sugar consumption, he also advises avoiding or reducing all products such as fruit juice or soft drinks. If you are thirsty, pure water is the best choice. Add a squeeze of lemon or lime juice for a little flavor. For more information on the C-SD visit siboinfo.com or gidoctor.net.

## SIBO BI-PHASIC DIET

The SIBO Bi-Phasic Diet is an offshoot of Dr. Siebecker's SIBO Specific Food Guide and the low-FODMAP diet. It was developed in 2013 by

Dr. Jacobi, who was seeking a more systematic approach for her SIBO patients, as many of them continued to react negatively to foods that were allowed in these diets. The SIBO Bi-Phasic Diet is designed to support a professional, individualized SIBO treatment plan, and is divided into two different phases. The first phase is called "reduce and repair" because it eliminates all carbohydrates that could potentially inflame the intestinal mucosa. This approach helps to remove stressful foods from the small intestine and initiate a self-healing process. This part of the "reduce and repair" phase may last several weeks. Dr. Jacobi emphasizes that a patient at this stage should receive an appropriate treatment plan, which may include dietary supplementation, remedies, and digestive support. The next step in this phase is a semi-restricted diet, which is introduced when symptoms have improved dramatically. Before beginning the second phase, "remove and restore", she recommends repeating a SIBO test to check whether the disease is still present. If the test result still shows SIBO, this second phase in the SIBO Bi-Phasic Diet can begin. During this phase bacteria are actively removed with an antimicrobial agent, with either an antibiotic or herbal product. At the same time, a prokinetic agent may be administered to restore gastrointestinal motility. Fortunately, during the first phase of the SIBO Bi-Phasic Diet bacteria have already been reduced, so that die-off reactions, such as fever, muscle aches, and headaches, are less severe now. Usually, the SIBO Bi-Phasic Diet takes about three months to complete. In severe cases it can take much longer. You can download a free PDF of this diet from Dr. Jacobi's educational The SIBO Doctor website.

If you are one of those people who tend to lose too much weight or don't get enough energy on other elimination diets, the SIBO Bi-Phasic Diet might be the right choice for you because it provides plenty of calories. Dr. Jacobi noticed that some clients, who were already on a restricted diet before treatment, developed symptoms that were due to nutrient deficiencies rather than SIBO. They often had difficulty reintroducing new foods. A very delicate situation.

Since the original SIBO Bi-Phasic Diet is very meat-heavy, many of Dr. Jacobi's patients wanted an alternative because they are either vegetarians, vegans, or just don't want to eat much of it. With this in mind, she developed a vegetarian version of the SIBO Bi-Phasic Diet in collaboration with Dr. Anne Criner, a naturopath and clinical nutritionist. Given that plant foods such as legumes can be difficult to digest, especially if the intestine is damaged, they have created an information sheet on soaking and sprouting methods to counteract this issue. They mentioned in the live launch of this new vegetarian diet on Facebook that a diet high in animal protein and saturated fat tends to produce inflammatory substances that stress the microbiome. This is especially true of animal products with high antibiotic content, as produced in modern livestock farming. A diet rich in plant food, on the other hand, provides plenty of polyphenols – antioxidants that have health-promoting properties. Dr. Criner explains that sprouting and soaking legumes as well as pseudo-grains like quinoa also helps to reduce FODMAPs, oxalates and salicylates. She advises adding legumes to your diet slowly, especially if you are not used to them. They are high in fiber and could aggravate symptoms. If they have been introduced into the diet, it is important to continue to consume these foods regularly even after a successful treatment. They are too beneficial to leave them out.

An easily digestible legume is the yellow split moong dahl, not to be confused with their green relatives, the mung beans. These still have their husk and can therefore cause digestive problems. In the Indian tradition, a dish called kicharee (or khichdi or kichari) is prepared for people with weak digestive systems. It is made of moong dahl and basmati rice with a little ghee and some spices such as cumin, coriander, fennel, and cinnamon. This simple one-pot solution can be eaten with seasonal vegetables or with a squeeze of lemon juice and some fresh cilantro. If you search the internet for the best way to prepare this dish, you'll find that there are as many recipes as there are cooks. Kicharee tastes best when freshly made and eaten straight away. Not only it is very good for the gut, but it also has a low GI, which keeps blood sugar levels stable. Moong dahl and basmati rice combined provide a complete protein, while the dahl provides additional magnesium. Fortunately, this dahl causes less flatulence than other legumes.

> I started soaking legumes, rice, nuts, seeds and pseudo grains a few years ago after attending a cooking demonstration by Chef Todd Stream Cameron featuring his cookbook *The Activated Grain Method. Easy, Nutritious & Delicious Gluten Free Recipes using The Activated Grain Method*. It's a great little book about legumes and other nutrient dense ingredients. It explains various techniques and background information on soaking, including recipes for breads, cakes, cookies and pancakes. I tried a few of them, and while not all recipes work equally well, I learned the basics of the process and can now easily create my own dishes. Since then, I like to have soaked grains in the fridge that I can use quickly.

## FAST TRACT DIET ™

The Fast Tract Diet was developed by Dr. Norm Robillard, a microbiologist, health expert, author, and the founder of the Digestive Health Institute, to help people with IBS and other digestive disorders. This diet evolved from his earlier work to find a treatment for GERD. Dr. Robillard, a GERD sufferer himself, was one of the first to suggest that excessive fermentation in the gastrointestinal tract is the underlying cause of acid reflux and restriction of carbohydrates can combat symptoms. Coming from the world of science, Dr. Robillard's approach is quite methodical. He developed a mathematical formula based on the fermentation potential (FP) of carbohydrates, their nutritional values and glycemic index. He says that eating lower FP carbohydrates allows for easier and faster digestion, and therefore better absorption of nutrients. The Fast Tract Diet is not limited to helping GERD patients, as it also helps people with digestive disorders such as SIBO, IBS, dysbiosis, leaky gut, celiac disease, Crohn's disease, ulcerative colitis, diverticulitis, asthma, and rosacea.

His FP rating system takes into account the symptom potential of each food and divides it into three categories – "low", "medium" and "high. If you want to manage your symptoms quickly, choose foods that have a low score. This diet does not exclude any food but pays attention to quantity. You may need to watch some foods more closely because they are generally harder to digest, such as resistant starch, fructose, fiber, and sugar alcohols (polyols). Interestingly, this system favors jasmine and sushi rice over basmati rice, even though these types of rice are very starchy, but still have a much lower FP.

To make the Fast Tract Diet more accessible for daily use, Dr. Robillard developed an app for iOS, iPad, and Android. It contains around 300 different foods with the option to add your own, create a shopping list, and monitor daily FP scores in relation to your symptoms. For more information, the app or a free FP calculator, visit his Digestive Health Institute website. For a more scientific view of this diet, check out his books: *Fast Tract Digestion: IBS. A Revolutionary Diet Approach to Treat and Prevent Irritable Bowel Syndrome* and *Fast Tract Digestion: Heartburn. A Revolutionary Diet System to Treat and Prevent Acid Reflux Without Drugs.*

## ELEMENTAL DIET

Back in the 1940s, scientists experimented with animals by giving them chemically formulated feeds containing simple and well-defined nutrients instead of food to analyze their growth, life, and reproduction. Based on these findings, studies were conducted to find a solution for people with nutrient deficiencies. Since then, various types of laboratory-prepared diets have been developed, each containing a predefined mixture of individual nutrients. One of the first uses of these elemental diets was for astronauts. On long missions, they were convenient, easy to store and produced little waste. During this era, the medical world adopted these types of diets in the clinical arena to support nutritional intake after surgery, especially for patients with Crohn's disease. Doctors realized that these diets not only improved patients' nutritional intake, but also led to remission of their diseases. Subsequently, the fields of application have expanded to inflammation-related diseases such as ulcerative colitis, eosinophilic esophagitis, cystic fibrosis, AIDS, acute pancreatitis, and rheumatic diseases, and the diet has also found its place in the treatment of SIBO, food allergies and intolerances.

The elemental diet is a dietary strategy for those who do not respond to other, conventional SIBO treatments, such as pharmaceutical or herbal antimicrobials, and is usually performed under medical supervision. The treatment requires a liquid diet in the form of a formula instead of solid food. The aim is to relieve the gastrointestinal tract and support its self-healing power. These formulas have sufficient calories, are easily digestible and provide essential macronutrients such as amino acids, simple sugars, minerals, vitamins, and fats - but lack fiber. They are absorbed primarily in the upper small intestine and allow inflammation to subside in the rest of the gastrointestinal tract. Unwanted bacteria are kept in check, allowing beneficial bacteria to colonize and provide a more balanced microbiome. The downside of the elemental diet is that it can promote fungal growth throughout the body, for example in the gut and mouth, and therefore requires special attention to counteract this phenomenon.

This diet has a success rate of about 80% in reducing gas production in the gastrointestinal tract within two to four weeks. Although not having to worry about food and happily sip on a yummy, flavored drink sounds quite tempting, it is anything but. Even though I have not tried the elemental diet myself (just a small sample, which was way too sweet for my taste and gave me diarrhea), I've heard that this diet is extremely regimented and most of the shakes taste terrible. Imagine drinking the same sweet chocolate drink all day long, perhaps for up to twenty days. According to reports from people who have done it, the first few days seem wonderful, but then it becomes increasingly harder to get the shake down. Not only do they struggle with not eating sold foods, but they also experience an emotional and physical roller coaster during this intense period.

Generally, it is recommended to repeat the SIBO test after fifteen days to see if there is still an overgrowth of bacteria in the small intestine. If the result is negative, you can stop the elemental diet and go into the post-treatment phase. However, if the result is not satisfactory, it is recommended to continue with the diet for a third week and then re-test. Again, if the result is still SIBO positive, you can continue the diet for a fourth week, or even longer in consultation with your healthcare provider. The post-treatment phase is primarily about getting the body used to proper solid foods again, which can be a lengthy process. So, it's not a good idea to go to your best friend's wedding right after the treatment and feast on the buffet – plan to have at least two months of just taking care of yourself. Even if you have done your best and gone through such a tough process, there is no guarantee that you will overcome SIBO for good. Do your research and read the stories of people who have made this journey. You'll find very different opinions on whether it was worth the effort. Rebecca Coomes (The Healthy Gut Podcast, episode 74, 2018) went through it. She gives many tips on how to prepare for this diet and what can happen during the process.

Make sure you are well informed before committing to the elemental diet, and if you do, don't plan on doing anything other than going through this procedure. Before you get too hard on yourself or think you must take on a burden to get healthy, think again. If you don't want to commit to the elemental diet in full, you can use a semi-elemental diet formula and have one or two shakes plus a light meal each day instead. This approach may be enough to achieve health improvements. Both versions of the elemental diet can be ordered through your healthcare provider. There is also a homemade recipe that can be found on Dr. Siebecker's website, that ends up being much cheaper than the store-bought varieties but doesn't necessarily taste any better. When you purchase a commercial product, make sure it doesn't contain whole proteins, corn, soy, gums, thickeners, preservatives, alcohol, or other foods that may affect your gastrointestinal system. You want to give your intestine the rest it needs and not irritate it even more with these ingredients. People who have Crohn's disease or colitis flare-ups often take these shakes for just a few days to relieve their symptoms. Other people use them to manage food allergies or to control their weight. Underweight people must pay special attention to sufficient caloric intake during the elemental diet, otherwise further health problems may occur. On the other hand, people belonging to this group can even benefit from this diet, because they get all the essential nutrients, and the calorie intake can be easily adjusted.

Due to the high sugar content of these formulas, they may not be suitable for diabetics. Another note of caution applies to those with impaired liver or kidney function, as the amino acid concentration in the shakes may affect these organs. If you have any concerns, please talk to your healthcare provider.

## NUTRITIONAL STRATEGY

I underwent an IgG food test in Germany. Along with my result, the company (ImuPro®) provided me with some additional information and recipes. Their approach to overcome inflammation and leaky gut is a dietary system divided into three phases. The first phase is to avoid all foods highlighted in the test result for five to eight weeks, as well as any foods that you already know cause symptoms. Within this time, a four-day rotational diet is implemented, which means that the food you eat on one day must be avoided on the following three days. In this way, food intolerances can be managed, and a varied and nutritious diet can be achieved. To keep track of what you have eaten, it is advisable to keep a food journal listing all ingredients including herbs, spices, and oils. In the provocation phase, new foods are introduced, either from the list or others that have been problematic for you. This is done slowly, one food at a time, three days apart, to make sure you catch any bodily responses. If you notice symptoms or a slight increase in body weight you should avoid the relevant foods again. Weight grain is caused by inflammatory responses triggered by these foods, followed by water retention in the intestine. This re-introduction procedure is carried out with all foods of concern; first all those that were labeled "moderate" on the test result, and then with those rated higher. The idea is that the immune system has time to forget that it had a problem with a particular food. Do not consume successfully reintroduced foods in excess; enjoy them perhaps once a week to avoid re-inflammation. Coffee and carbonated drinks are irritants to the gut, so do not consume them, or if you must, alternate them like other foods. Soft drinks in particular cause health problems because they can bind calcium and prevent the body from utilizing important minerals. Alcoholic beverages are also on the "no-no" list of this diet.

Another insight I gained from the company's information material concerns the issue of allergens and cross-reaction. For example, if you react to latex, it is likely that you will also have issues with pineapples, melons, bananas, and contact with the houseplant Benjamin fig. All have similar allergens. Another example is ginger and walnut, both of which have the same allergenic structure as birch pollen. Sensitivity to mugwort pollen can also lead to problems with nutmeg, and so forth. The list is endless, and if you are not a specialist in this field it is not easy to keep track.

## AUTOIMMUNE PALEO DIET

It is scientifically recognized that dietary changes can improve the microbiome and our health. This is where the Autoimmune Paleo diet

(AIP) comes in. It not only stops the body's self-attack, but also supports the healing of damaged tissues, reduces inflammation, regulates hormones, heals leaky gut and creates a healthy microbiome. The AIP is built on nutrient-dense foods derived equally from animals and plants. It omits many ingredients such as grains, pseudo-grains like amaranth and quinoa, legumes, sugars, nuts and seeds, nightshade vegetables, as well as all processed foods.

This strict diet is not for the faint-hearted but for many it is the last resort to regain their health. Some may be able to reverse their auto-immune disease with this dietary approach, while others may need to follow AIP or a similar approach for the rest of their lives to achieve a reasonable quality of life. Dr. Ballantyne is a well-known advocate of this diet and has written a fantastic book called *The Paleo Approach. Reverse Autoimmune Disease and Heal Your Body*. Another like-minded author is Dr. Terry Wahls, who wrote *The Wahls Protocol. A Radical New Way to Treat All Chronic Autoimmune Conditions Using Paleo Principles*. Both authors explain in detail why their nutrition approach can help to reverse autoimmune disease.

## WHOLE30

The Whole30 is a modified and restricted Paleo diet. This elimination diet was developed in 2009 by husband-and-wife team Melissa and Dallas Hartwig to promote a better physical and emotional relationship with food. In their book *The Whole30: The 30-Day Guide to Total Health and Food Freedom*, they point the finger particularly at comfort foods, why we become addicted to them, and how we can leave cravings behind. They note that the scientific background of this diet is detailed in their book *It Starts with Food: Discover the Whole30 and Change Your Life in Unexpected Ways*.

The Whole30 is an anti-inflammatory diet that has the side effect of weight loss. It is claimed that if you follow the protocol, you will most likely have more energy, healthy digestion, better sleep, and improved mood. Participants report improvements in many lifestyle-related diseases and conditions such as asthma, high blood pressure, cholesterol, migraine, depression, joint pain, IBS, and leaky gut. Although this is not a classic SIBO and IBS diet, I mention it because it can help you develop a different perspective on food, especially reward foods and snacks. As the name implies, it is a thirty-day diet that avoids foods such as sugar - including honey - all grains, dairy, legumes, processed foods, and alcohol. Cheating or slipping is not allowed, or you will have to start all over again. Once completed, foods are slowly reintroduced to see if you have issues with any of them. This diet is supported by a large community. You can get involved in social media groups, hire a coach, and buy one of the many cookbooks from different authors.

## THE MEDITERRANEAN STYLE DIET

The Mediterranean style diet is an eating pattern based on the traditional cuisines of Greece, Italy and other countries bordering the Mediterranean Sea. It is highly praised in the scientific world for its health benefits and considered one of the healthiest and most sustainable dietary models in the world. Numerous studies show that a Mediterranean style diet positively affects the microbiome, meaning also the digestive and immune systems. It can help reduce inflammation of the intestinal mucosa - a condition that occurs for instance in IBS - and can counteract oxidative stress. At the same time this diet reduces the risk of heart diseases and cognitive decline, which is associated with dementia and Alzheimer's disease. The Mediterranean style diet even has the potential to reverse metabolic syndromes and type 2 diabetes. An advocate of this dietary approach is Dr. Mosley, a British science journalist and author of numerous books. He developed several diet programs such as the 5:2 diet, Fast 800 and Fast 800 Keto, all based on the Mediterranean style diet, to help others overcome weight gain, obesity and type 2 diabetes. His mission is a personal one, as he himself was diagnosed with type 2 diabetes but was able to successfully reverse this disease with diet and exercises.

Plant-based foods such as whole grains, vegetables, fruits, legumes, nuts, seeds, herbs and spices are the foundation of the Mediterranean style diet. Preferred are locally produced foods that are in season. This diet is complemented by moderate consumption of fish and other sea-foods or some poultry, eggs and dairy products, but has a very low amounts of red meat, refined carbohydrate, and sweets. Olive oil is the predominant added fat. Daily intake of adequate water and physical activities are strongly recommended. People in the Mediterranean regions enjoy sharing meals with loved ones - which adds a social component that is health promoting on a whole different level.

Although this diet is very healthy, you should not overdo it. Overeating can lead to weight gain. Focusing on a balanced food plate, as recommended by the Harvard T.H. Chan School of Public Health, can be a helpful guide here. According to them, half of the plate should consist of vegetables and some fruits, a quarter of whole grain products and, as a maximum, a quarter of protein-containing foods.

> The bottom line of all the diets presented here is that they have the potential to relieve bothersome symptoms in a short period of time and bring aware-ness to the quality and quantity of food we eat. During the dieting there were many moments when I would have normally reached for processed foods, treats and snacks. After being confronted about my eating habits, I was determined to change them. Today, I no longer feel the need to bake a cupcake, eat pizza, or eat sweets, not even the "healthy" versions. Some of the above diets have their limitations, as they do not provide long-term dietary variety. They can even promote an eating disorder, as sufferers are afraid to reintroduce foods and stay on a restricted diet for too long. Person-ally, I stick to the Mediterranean diet offered by Dr. Mosley. It is delicious, varied and healthy. Along with some Ayurvedic wisdom, it has helped me relieve symptoms such as bloating.

# AYURVEDA

After several years of following protocol after protocol, I was able to get SIBO and IBS under control and yet felt quite stressed by the regime I was subjecting myself to. My healthcare provider didn't have much more up her sleeve for further improvement than to offer me the elemental diet. That's when I began to wonder if I was on the right path. Couldn't it be more harmful to my body and soul to live constantly in a state of self-restraint? Why did I develop these diseases? Why does everything jam up in the center of my body? What am I holding on to and why are the natural movements in my intestines stagnating? The conclusion I drew from these thoughts reinforced my decision to no longer go the medical and naturopathic path for these diseases. My quest was to find an holistic approach for my body and mind that I could easily integrate into my life without stressing my nervous system – so I came to Ayurveda.

To this day, traditional medicines remain an integral part of many cultures. Some countries adopt them and call them "complementary medicine" because they are not part of their own tradition or medical system. Dr. Margaret Chan, Director-General of WHO says that for millions of people, herbal medicines, traditional treatments, and practitioners are the main source of health care, if not the only source. She emphasizes that they are accessible and affordable and "stand out as a way of coping with the relentless rise of chronic non-communicable diseases". Like almost all traditional medicines, Ayurveda has a long history of preventing and treating diseases. It is a medical system based on the idea that diseases are caused by an imbalance or stress in the human being. Along with yoga, it was developed several millennia ago to help people live a lifestyle that supports the maintenance of health and the prevention and cure of diseases. Ayurveda is a Sanskrit term for ayur (life) and veda (knowledge). In the early days of Ayurveda, highly respected, intellectual, and spiritual persons were given the comprehensive task of creating a medical system that would alleviate human suffering and serve humanity. Later, in the Hindu tradition of the sixth century BC, a compilation of details providing a systematic approach to all types of medical issues, treatments and wellness was recorded. These first scientific works were refined and expanded over several centuries to include various fields such as internal medicine, psychology, pediatrics, and surgery. The fact that the Ayurvedic system is still practiced today is probably because it focuses on the inherent causes of a disease and not so much on its external influences. Civilization and human habits may have changed in the millennia since this system was first introduced, but man's responses to disease, such as signs and symptoms, are still the same as that of our ancestors.

Long before modern science recognized the importance of the relationship between the mind and the gut for human wellbeing, Ayurveda had assumed that all diseases originate in the mind and can strongly affect the digestive system. This symbiotic connection allows the disease to be approached from different angles, whether from the mind and/or the gut. Ayurvedic practitioners often address the gut first, focusing on improving digestive and metabolic functions and strengthening the immune system. Later, they may provide advice on how to address any mental imbalance.

Ayurveda is not a quick fix to get well. Instead, it aims to make changes in a person's life to create a physical and mental balance to resist and cure disease. Due to its Eastern terminology and philosophical principles, understanding Ayurveda may be challenging at first. To Western ears, it can be quite bewildering when a practitioner talks about agni, ama, doshas, and ojas, and uses hard-to-pronounce names for remedies and treatments. It may also take some time to get used to the five-element theory (earth, water, fire, air, and space), which corresponds to our five senses and is the basis of the Ayurvedic philosophy. Despite this, do not be discouraged because even small applications of Ayurvedic wisdom can make a difference in your life. Perhaps you like to try their food combination to support optimal gastrointestinal tract function? According to Ayurveda, certain combinations of foods aggravate diseases, while others promote health. Kester Marshall, owner and Ayurvedic practitioner at the Mudita Institute in Australia says fruit should always be eaten alone and spaced apart from other foods; an exception may be made if it is cooked. The reason it is best to consume it separately is that fresh fruit is usually somewhat acidic and therefore digested more quickly. When it is combined with more complex and alkaline foods, there is a significant discrepancy between their fermentation times, which creates a conflict situation in the body that causes symptoms such as gas and bloating.

In Ayurveda, food is medicine, and it is important to develop a basic understanding of what you eat, as well as when and how you eat. It is recommended to eat at a similar time each day, with a modest breakfast, a larger filling lunch (when the "digestive fire" is the strongest), and a light dinner such as a soup or some steamed vegetables, if needed at all. Ayurveda also advises leaving enough time for fasting between meals so that the digestive system can do its cleansing work before new food comes along. This is the same approach I explained in the section on the MMC. Eating in a quiet and relaxed environment is vital, as anger, fear and upset can lead to a dysregulation of the metabolism. Constant arguing, hectic or other negative influences during meals can cause chronic diseases such as gastritis, stomach ulcers, and IBS.

One of the main characteristics of an Ayurvedic way of eating is to support the different physical and mental constitutions (doshas). There are three main dosha types: vata, pitta, and kapha. Most people fall into a combination or mix of these body types, such as vata-pitta, pitta-kapha, or vata-kapha, with one of them usually dominating. You can eat according to your body type, but don't make a religion out of this way of eating, because it only leads to unnecessary stress. It's just a guide for you to shimmy along. Although an Ayurvedic way of eating does not usually have specific dietary restrictions, it is predominantly vegetarian and emphasizes fresh ingredients to create light, warm cooked meals with a slightly oily touch. Herbs and spices are an essential part of this diet, as they enhance digestion and metabolism, remove accumulated food waste, and have therapeutic value for various parts of the body. For example, ginger can help with gas and bloating and is also a good remedy for nausea and respiration issues. Turmeric is known as an anti-inflammatory agent. Cumin relieves chest congestion; and fennel water can bring relief to a colicky baby – and its parents, too.

> One of my favorite home remedies for upset stomach (but not limited to this application) is a blend of five digestive spices. For this remedy, you need to mix fennel, coriander, cumin and cardamom seeds and ginger powder in equal parts, preferably organic, and grind the mix. Keep it in a small container, and if needed, take a teaspoon and mix it with about 50 ml of hot water. Wait until it cools down and drink it. Don't worry, you don't have to drink the stuff that settled at the bottom of the glass. This remedy speeds up the motility of the bowels and quickly helps with cramps. I have tried it a few times and was amazed at how quickly the relief came. I always have some at home or with me when I travel.

If you are interested in an Ayurvedic approach to improving your health and don't know where to start, Dr Douillard's Lifespa website is a helpful resource with its free and comprehensive information. Of course, there are many other websites dedicated to Ayurveda. Or, you may simply want to book a consultation with an Ayurvedic practitioner. An Ayurvedic practitioner observes a patient thoroughly, takes the pulse in a certain way and checks the tongue. The treatment may include herbal remedies, enemas, massages, dietary changes or even fasting. But don't worry if the latter has been suggested to you, it doesn't mean you have to go hungry. Rather, it is about eating lighter meals that are suitable for your constitution or current state of health. It gives your digestive system a break and helps eliminate accumulated substances in the body, which strengthens the digestive system to prepare for the metabolism of heavy and indigestible foods. A tailored diet and use of herbal remedies to restore an imbalanced digestive system are especially effective for dysbiosis, SIBO, and IBS. Quite often the nervous system is somewhat tense under these health conditions. Calming can be achieved through the regular application of an Abhyanga self-massage, which is also excellent for improving blood circulation, joint lubrication, and lymphatic drainage. For a restful sleep, it should be done in the evening, while a morning massage provides a good start to the day. This warm, oily self-massage is easy to perform. Depending on person's dosha, different oils are used to support individual needs. There are many practical tips and information on the internet on how to perform this massage or let an Ayurvedic practitioner explain it to you.

You may think that Ayurveda is not the right path for you if you have digestive problems because it seems so different from the Western approach; or you may be put off by the spiritual approach of the Maharishi movement in the 1970s and 1980s. Nonetheless, you may want to reconsider. Faced with rising health care costs and helplessness in dealing with these diseases, people are seeking to take their healing into their own hands. To meet this challenge, traditional medicine with its long history and experience in health care is certainly worth considering. You may already be familiar with some of the practices that are integrated and accepted in Western culture, such as acupuncture, chiropractic, homeopathy, naturopathy, and osteopathy. Not only are they often more affordable, especially in countries where they are deeply rooted in culture and history, but they also underscore the importance of individualized, person-centered care. This is all the truer because alternative practitioners often compensate for the lack of dialogue between patients and doctors in Western-oriented medicine. Getting enough attention to talk about one's compromised health and the stresses associated with it promotes mental health – an important component of recovery.

A word of caution. Like all dietary supplements, traditional medicine products are not subject to the official drug regulatory system. Some of these products may interact with conventional medicines, so you need to consult your doctor before consumption. Please do not use products that may be of poor quality, adulterated or counterfeit, as they pose a health risk. Before consulting a complementary practitioner, whether from Ayurveda or another discipline, take the time to inform yourself about their training and practices to avoid disappointment. There is a wide range of qualifications on the market, and not all of them are trustworthy. Women who are pregnant or breastfeeding, as well as children, should first see a doctor before going to a traditional healer.

I consider myself very fortunate to have an excellent Ayurvedic practitioner. Not only does he have a wealth of knowledge, but his consultation fees are very reasonable compared to other consultations I have used in the past. Every treatment or recommendation he gives me is designed to improve my health in the long term. It may not be the fastest way to see results, but it is certainly the easiest for me so far. I don't feel overwhelmed by his recommendations or the Ayurvedic diet, which allows me to focus on more enjoyable things in my life as my condition continues to improve.

# SEASONAL EATING

Seasonal eating is an integral part of Ayurveda and another effective way to build a healthy microbiome. The term "seasonal", distinguishes between global and local seasonal produce. Seasonal produce grown for global distribution is typically harvested when immature, stored for an extended period of time, and transported to other countries around the world, ensuring a varied and constant supply of fresh produce throughout the year. The disadvantage of this system is that the produce is mostly grown in agricultural monocultures, which leads to the loss of species and crops, as well as ecological biodiversity. You may have heard that insect populations round the world have declined dramatically. Although many consider them pests, they play an important role in the ecological health of the planet, as many animals and plants depend on them. A reason for this loss of insects is the impact of modern agriculture on their habitats and its use of pesticides and fertilizers.

An alternative to eating produce grown in monocultures is to eat food grown within your climate zone. This local, seasonal produce is sold mainly in the respective region of the country. It is harvested when ripe and is transported only a short distance to reach the consumer. A smaller agricultural industry allows for greater biodiversity, supports the local economies, and enables direct contact with the consumer. By growing your own food, buying it at the farmer's market or from your local farmer, you not only reduce plastic packaging and transportation, but also reduce your carbon footprint and contribute to the fight against climate change.

We are closely connected to the biodiversity of our region and our bodies adapt much better to various conditions when we eat seasonal, local products. The microbiology of the soil changes with the seasons and so do the microorganisms in our microbiome. Dr. Douillard is a strong supporter of local and seasonal produce as it boosts beneficial microbes in the microbiome and contributes to overall health. This fact is confirmed by scientists who studied the stool of the Hadza hunters and gatherers in Tanzania. They found that this tribe develops specific enzymes for foods that are only available at certain times of the year. Interestingly, some of their microbes disappear altogether in other seasons, only to reappear later on. The researchers discovered that this biological process allows a much better utilization of the consumption of plant-based carbohydrates. When this study compared Hadza people with healthy Westerners, they also found seasonal changes in the microbiome of the latter group. However, it is limited and less diverse.

In most Western countries, we are spoiled by having fresh food available all year round. Something is always in season somewhere, and it can be tricky to know what is regional and what is not. You can check the labels of the fresh food at your grocer that may indicate the country of origin. For example, you might find grapes and kiwi fruit from overseas. The online Seasonal Food Guide Australia provides a list of foods and indicates which is in season in which region in Australia. For the US, it is worth checking out the Food Print website as it provides comprehensive information on sustainable shopping and eating, as well as a great seasonal food guide app for Mac iOS and Android.

To cure or prevent gastrointestinal diseases, you can rely on a healthy diet with lots of fresh ingredients – creating a diverse microbiome that in return keeps diseases away. The Stanford University microbiologist Justin Sonnenburg, who led the Hadza Tanzania study, says: "Humans are not just a collection of cells. We are composite organisms. Just like ecosystems – like a rainforest composed of thousands of species. We need all of the species to work in concert for us to be healthy".

# THE ART OF EATING

Since we were children, we unconsciously observed everything that revolved around food in our environment, and this went far beyond tasting it. While our caregivers mostly organized when and what we should eat, and sometimes how much, there are subtle feelings associated with meals. Did your mother have an aversion to cooking, or did she embrace it to the point that it was her sole domain? Was your father involved in the kitchen? Did you experience the dining table as a battlefield or a silent event? Maybe you didn't even have a set routine and an assigned place to eat, and grew up like a free-range chicken that could pop something in its mouth at will. Whatever you experienced and perceived, it most likely shaped your relationship with food today. When it comes to food, you are probably dependent on many external circumstances, such as your job and family. Bakeries, canteens, food courts, and restaurants are often the mainstays of catering. Few of us bother to cook for ourselves every day, especially when there is no family to feed. A quick breakfast on the run, a small lunch – maybe a salad because you don't want to feel too heavy afterwards – and a hearty dinner that has enough carbohydrates to fill you up after a long day. If you add the many snacks between meals, you get the picture of typical modern eating habits. Please believe me, I used to eat the same way and thought I had a healthy diet.

The omnipresent compulsion to feed our bodies on a regular basis drives us to be constantly on the lookout for food. No question, the right diet fulfills an important aspect in our lives, for it can promote health. For my taste, however, our relationship with food is a little out of hand these days. I have the impression that we live in a pop culture in which chefs and food play the starring roles. Not only should food taste, look and smell fantastic but also entertain us. We watch countless food demonstrations on television, attend live food events, buy food magazines and books, or search the Internet for the latest recipes. These influences go so far that it seems individual, isolated "superfoods" should increase our performance and make us healthy.

If one searches for an answer that explains what healthy eating is, one comes across numerous scientific studies, theories, views, and teachings that propagate guidelines for the "right" diet, with almost everything represented from strict asceticism to excess. The bottom line is that a healthy diet maintains and improves overall health by providing the body with essential nutrients, fluids, and sufficient calories. To pass this message on to the population, the nutrition societies of the respective countries issue dietary guidelines to try to prevent various forms of malnutrition. These guidelines are usually presented in the form of an illustrated pyramid or a plate. In these illustrations, foods are divided into groups with certain nutritional properties, each of which can be consumed in certain amounts to ensure a balanced diet. These guidelines have evolved over the years and will continue to do so as more knowledge about nutrition is gained. Scientists have now realized that counting calories or joules may not be enough if you want to lose weight, but that you should also pay attention to the quality of the food you eat. That's why the term "nutrient-dense" foods is popping up in the media, which describes the amount of beneficial nutrients in a food relative to its calories, weight, and harmful components. Daily consumption of these high-quality foods supports the absorption of needed nutrients and thus overall health.

For a better understanding, nutrients are divided into macronutrients and micronutrients. Macronutrients are proteins, fats and carbohydrates that serve as energy sources for the body. While micronutrients are associated with the "nutrient-dense" foods mentioned above. They contain important components such as amino acids, vitamins, minerals, and trace elements, from which no energy can be obtained but which are essential for the functions of our body. If you want to know which foods belong to this category, you can check out Dr. Fuhrman's website.

He is a board-certified family physician, author and nutrition expert who offers the Aggregate Nutrient Density Index (ANDI), a list of the most common foods in this group. Another source of information on this topic is the study *"Uncovering the Nutritional Landscape of Food"* by Kim, S., et. al., 2015. At the bottom of this study, you'll find two downloadable data sets (S1 and S2), both include hundreds of foods.

When buying food, try to buy fresh organic produce which is more likely to provide more nutrients because it is grown in a healthier soil. At the same time, you support sustainable agriculture. Purchasing and preparing fresh ingredients is like a prelude to digestion, as our senses of touch, smell, sight, and taste help initiate full readiness. Although we like to rely on information and nutritional insights from research and media reports, it's important to remember that there are no universal guidelines when it comes to metabolism, meaning factors such as genes, age, culture, and lifestyle strongly influence this process. After all, we are too individual to take generalizations about nutrition too seriously.

A healthy diet is not the only way to make a personal contribution to our wellbeing. Before focusing solely on *what* to eat, we should also consider *how* we eat. I mentioned earlier in the chapter on stress that it is desirable to calm the nervous system, so that body functions can operate optimally. My best advice is don't eat when you are in a hurry or feeling tense. Find a comfortable, relaxed environment and eat more slowly. Don't shovel food into yourself; instead, take your time while eating. Pause between each bite so that oxygen gets into your body through gentle breathing. Be mindful of what you eat and where it has come from. Let every bite be a feast. Your body will thank you because you are giving it time to properly analyze the incoming food so that it can distribute its nutrients where they are needed most. This way of eating not only contributes to a healthy body weight, but also to healthy bone structure. Stop eating when you are comfortably full, no matter how delicious the food is.

Researchers have recognized that it is very important to maintain an eating rhythm that is synchronized with our circadian rhythm. The circadian rhythm is a natural, internal process that regulates the sleep-wake rhythm and repeats itself approximately every 24 hours. This rhythm is linked to our biological clocks, which regulate the timing of bodily processes. Environmental influences and lifestyle - including light exposure, sleep patterns, temperature, physical activity, social interaction, and mealtimes – can correlate with the circadian rhythm and may affect the functions of these internal clocks.

Three American scientists, Jeffrey C. Hall, Michael Rosbash and Michael W. Young, discovered two new genes that control circadian rhythms during their research on fruit flies, which earned them the Nobel Prize in 2017. The period gene accumulates a protein in the cells at night and degrades during the day. The timeless gene, on the other hand, controls the biological clocks of the cells.The synchronization and the mechanism of these two genes strongly influence cells, the brain and almost every organ system, including the digestive tract and metabolism. Any disturbance that causes the central clock and peripheral clocks to become out of sync results in altered tissue structure and functions that can lead to long-term organ damage. Researchers have linked this condition to various gastrointestinal disorders, such as IBS, inflammatory bowel disease, GERD, impaired motility and microbiome, as well as accelerated aging and cancer.

When we work against our biological clocks by turning day into night and vice versa, we disrupt the production of the hormone melatonin, which is produced in the pineal gland and released at night to help us fall asleep. The gastrointestinal tract requires a considerable amount of melatonin to protect the mucosa and prevent conditions such as leaky gut. Melatonin also acts as an antioxidant, promotes blood circulation, and has immune-regulating functions. Irregular sleep patterns are not the only cause of disturbed melatonin production. The same applies to environmental factors such as too much or the wrong light in the evenings, lack of exercise, and too little social contacts. I have already discussed all these issues in previous chapters. Just as important is when we eat our meals. As part of the 24-hour cycle, our body expects certain forms of energy from food at certain times of the day. Scientists have found that digestion works best when we eat the most calories in the first half of the day when the sun is at its highest. They also found that skipping breakfast and eating a meal after 3 p.m. can lead to weight gain and to negative changes in the microbiome. These eating habits, including regular snacking, are closely linked to IBS, appetite disorder, and sleep disorders. If you regularly eat late at night, glucose tolerance worsens, and metabolic rhythm is disrupted. It is known that irregular or drastic changes in eating habits, possibly related to work schedules or travel abroad, may also be a cause of obesity, type 2 diabetes, and cardiovascular disease.

Ayurveda places special emphasis on biorhythms and daily routines. When these routines are followed, they promote stability and a sense of grounding, calming the nervous system and supporting bodily functions. It is said that the body is in deep resonance with recurring cycles, as the internal organs and tissues know when to prepare and what to expect. This traditional medical system is based on the principle that nature regulates the inside and outside of the body. For this reason, the doshas are assigned not only to the human body, but also to different times of the day. A 24-hour cycle in Ayurveda is divided into four hourly periods, each corresponding to one of the doshas. The phase around midday belongs to the pitta dosha, the "king of digestion" – a hot, sharp, fiery energy that gives the body strength to process a substantial meal. In the afternoon, the light, dry, airy vata dosha predominates. To balance this energy, a warm and slightly oily snack is recommended, such as warm milk with a little ghee or butter, perhaps also something soothing like nut butter, herbal tea or just warm water. Do not reach out in the afternoon for typical snacks such as crackers, chips, popcorn, cookies, dried fruit and don't overindulge in raw vegetables, as all of these aggravates vata and can make you feel nervous, anxious, tired, and bloated. To end the day harmoniously, dinner should be eaten by 6 p.m. at best, but no later than 8 p.m., as vata changes to the kapha dosha. This is an earthy, cool, and energetically rather heavy dosha that needs a moderate, warm and light meal such as a soup or steamed vegetables to balance it. The Ayurvedic cycle continues with a resurgence of pitta dosha at 10 p.m., which uses its power to aid digestion during the night, and vata dosha at 2 a.m. to assist with elimination. At sunrise, the cycle continues as the kapha dosha re-emerges to prepare the metabolism for the day. Again, a warm, light meal between 6 a.m. and 10 a.m. can balance its heavy nature.

Even though Western and Eastern cultures seem so different, they are not, because both serve humanity by systematically observing circumstances and drawing conclusions from them. Each of them has awakened in me an understanding of what I may need to be healthy. Whichever way you choose, try to find the root cause of your gut problem. Don't settle for solutions that only help in the short term, because you may soon find yourself in the same situation again. Take one step at a time and find out what your body and mind truly need and how you can accommodate it. It is worth it, because the body is the companion to life.

# CONCEPT SUMMARY

» Certain types of grains contain proteins that form gluten when they come into contact with water. This glue-like substance is great for baking, but can cause health problems for some people and severely affect digestion. This is especially true for people with celiac disease, and also more or less for people who do not have this disease but are still sensitive to gluten.

» Oats are naturally gluten-free, but can cause health issues similar to those caused by gluten. The reason for this is that it is often grown in the vicinity of gluten-containing grains and processed in the same machinery. Cross-contamination may not be the only reason for bodily complaints, because oats also contain FODMAPs and the oat protein can be difficult to digest, and it is rich in fiber.

» Diets for IBS and SIBO are of different origins and vary in their approaches. Overall, they aim to relieve symptoms by eliminating certain foods from the diet. These diets should not be followed for a long period of time, as they may lack nutritional diversity.

» Traditional medicine such as Ayurveda has a valued place in healthcare. This system promotes dietary and lifestyle practices to prevent or treat disease. Its treatment approach to gastrointestinal disorders and non-communicable diseases is a valuable complement to modern medicine.

» Seasonal, local produce establishes a natural connection to the region we live in, leading to a more adaptable gut microbiome. Each of these foods, influenced by the season and the composition of the soil, provides specific enzymes and nutrients that are tailored to our bodies.

» We are part of a solar rhythm that affects the Earth and our bodies. It is not enough to focus on what we eat, but also how and when we eat. Science, and traditional medicine such as Ayurveda are largely in agreement on this matter.

# DEAR READER

Thank you so much for your interest in this book! If you've found it valuable, I would be incredibly grateful if you could share your thoughts in a review on platforms like Amazon, Barnes & Noble, or any other sites you prefer. Your feedback is crucial—it helps other readers discover my book and supports them on their journey to better health. Your contribution truly makes a difference!

Before you close this book, I'd love to stay connected with you. Visit my website at www.mygut.com, where you can subscribe to my newsletter, find my social media accounts, or just drop me a message. I look forward to staying in touch and continuing this journey together!

# ACKNOWLEDGMENTS

I am very grateful to all those who helped me to bring this book to life with their heart, soul and time, particularly as English is not my first language. Many thanks go to Ashni and Majjham for helping me revise the first drafts. To my editors Heather Miller and Ellen Ward. Without Ellen's call for clarity, support, and encouragement, this book would not have reached its maturity. To Kate Theobald for her beautiful textile artwork that shines on the cover of this book.

To my very beloved mother who sadly passed away all too early. To my sisters, who are far away but very dear to me, and whom I often thought of when I wrote, especially on subjects that might be of interest to them. To all my friends who have supported me with their words of encouragement to not give up, and to finish this book. To my wonderful boys and husband for their support, endless patience and trust in me.

I would like to thank all the professional healthcare providers and mentors who have supported me on my health journey, especially to Dr. Annette Beisenherz, Dr. Marcus Hewitson, Dr. Nirala Jacobi, Sonya Cacciotti and Dr. Michael Hayter. Thanks to Sarita Ford for all the laughter in our hypnosis sessions. To Kester Marshall for your Ayurvedic wisdom. To Fara Curlewis and Marilette Liongson for making Master Choa Kok Sui's teachings accessible to me.

A special thank you also goes to Dr. Mark Pimentel, Dr. Allison Siebecker, and Shivan Sarna and the many others who work tirelessly to educate the public about IBS and SIBO.

If I have forgotten anyone who contributed to the creation and success of this book, please forgive me and, thank you!

# GLOSSARY

**ACHLORHYDRIA**
A condition that occurs when the stomach has no hydrochloric acid, an essential component of gastric acid. Achlorhydria is associated with a deficiency of vitamins and minerals such as vitamins C and D, folic acid, and iron.

**ADRENAL FATIGUE SYNDROME**
A collection of non-specific symptoms often associated with poor stress response, digestive problems, fatigue, sleep disturbances, and cravings for salty and sweet foods.

**ALPHA-LACTALBUMIN**
A whey protein found in the milk of almost all mammalian species. It plays an important role in the synthesis of lactose.

**AMINO ACIDS**
Organic compounds made up of nitrogen, carbon, hydrogen, and oxygen that make up proteins. Amino acids are essential for our bodies and some of them must be supplied through diet as we can't synthesize them ourselves.

**AMYGDALA**
A region in the brain primarily associated with emotional processes.

**ANEMIA**
A condition that results from a lack of red blood cells, which are responsible for carrying oxygen to the body's tissues. There are several types of anemia, with iron deficiency being a common one.

**ANTI-INFLAMMATORY**
A property of a substance or treatment that counteracts or relieves inflammation, pain, and swelling.

**ANTIBIOTIC**
A medication used to treat infections or diseases caused by bacteria.

**ANTIGEN**
Foreign macromolecules that react with the cells of the immune system, triggering the immune response.

**ANTIMICROBIAL**
An active agent, either of natural or pharmaceutical origin, for example herb or antibiotic, which eliminates microorganisms or stops their growth.

**ANTIOXIDANT**
Any substance, either of natural or synthetic origin that can prevent or slow down damage to cells from oxidation.

**ANTI-NUTRIENT**
Any substance, either of natural or synthetic origin that interferes with the absorption of nutrients.

**APOPTOSIS**
A highly controlled form of cell death, akin to cell suicide, to eliminate unwanted cells in the body.

**ARABINOXYLAN**
A type of cellulose that is found in the outer shell of plants including wood and grains such as wheat, rye, oats, and rice.

**ARCHAEA**
An ancient microorganism that shapes life on earth.

**ASPERGILLOSIS**
An infection caused by a type of mold or fungus that affects the respiration system.

**AUTOIMMUNE DISEASE**
A condition in which the autoimmune system mistakenly attacks the body's own cells, tissues, or organs.

**AUTONOMIC NERVOUS SYSTEM**
A branch of the peripheral nervous system that regulates the functions of internal organs and muscles.

**BASEMENT MEMBRANE**
A thin, sheet-like matrix that provides support for epithelial cells and serves as a boundary to the underlying connective tissue. It can also influence the behavior of the cells.

**BETA CELLS**
Specialized cells in the pancreas that produce, store, and release the hormone insulin to facilitate the absorption of glucose.

**BETA-LACTOGLOBULIN**
A whey protein found abundantly in milk

**BETAINE HYDROCHLORIDE**
A chemical substance, either natural or synthetic in origin that may be helpful in a deficiency of gastric acid production.

**BIFIDOBACTERIUM**
A group of gram-positive bacteria that live in the mammalian microbiome, also a common component of probiotics.

**BILE**
A digestive fluid produced in the liver and stored in the gallbladder, and carried to the small intestine to aid digestion.

**BIOFEEDBACK THERAPY**
A technology that can both measure and subtly alter physiological functions by using sensors attached to the body.

**BIOFILM**
An accumulation of various microorganisms adhered to a surface.

**BIOMARKERS**
Biological properties or molecules that indicate and allow biological states or conditions to be evaluated.

**BIOTIN**
An essential nutrient that converts food into energy, also known as vitamin B7.

**BLOOD SUGAR (GLUCOSE) LEVEL**
A measure of the concentration of glucose in the blood.

**BODY MASS INDEX**
A measure of body fat based on height and weight to categorize weight ranges.

**BRAIN FOG**
Not a medical or scientific term, describes a condition where a person lacks mental clarity and is unable to concentrate.

**BUTYRATE**
An SCFA produced by gut microbes when they metabolize dietary fiber.

**CANDIDA (CANDIDIASIS)**
A fungal infection caused by yeast.

**CECUM**
A pouch in the first part of the large intestine that acts as a reservoir for chyme.

**CELIAC DISEASE**
An immune reaction to the gluten protein that is present in certain types of grains, such as wheat, barley, and rye.

**CENTRAL NERVOUS SYSTEM**
Consists of the brain and spinal cord and plays a 'central' role in most bodily functions.

**CHRONIC FATIGUE**
A chronic, complex, and prolonged disease that is characterized by extreme fatigue and tiredness, pain, memory loss, or lack of concentration.

**CHYME**
A thick acidic liquid containing gastric juices and partially digested semi-liquid mass that is passes from the stomach into the small intestine.

**CIRCADIAN RHYTHM**
A rhythm set by the environment, mainly by the solar day, to which the body's own processes adapt.

**CLOSTRIDIUM**
A gram-positive, anaerobic bacteria found in the environment and the gastrointestinal tract of humans and other animals that can cause food poisoning and infections.

**COGNITIVE THERAPY**
Structured psychotherapy that addresses inaccurate or negative thinking and assists a person to act and respond more effectively in challenging situations.

**COLECTOMY**
A surgical procedure that removes all or parts of the colon.

**COLLAGEN**
An abundant protein that provides strength and structure in the body and is found in the connective tissue of mammals.

**COLONOSCOPY**
An endoscopic examination used to examine and diagnose bowel diseases. For this purpose, a small camera at the end of a flexible tube is inserted through the rectum

**COLONY FORMING UNITS**
A method to measure a sample of microbes such as bacteria and fungi on a petri plate.

**COLOSTRUM**
The first form of milk produced after birth, which contains protective properties for the baby.

**CORONARY CALCIUM SCAN**
A special cardiac exam that uses a CT scan to evaluate the amount of calcium present in relation to the risk of a heart attack.

**CORONARY HEART DISEASE**
A heart condition that occurs when large blood vessels are blocked, damaged, or diseased.

**CORTISOL**
A steroid hormone produced by the adrenal glands widely known as the body's stress hormone.

**CROHN'S DISEASE**
A chronic, incurable, and painful inflammatory bowel disease characterized by inflammation of the digestive tract.

**CYST**
An abnormally grown nodular pocket filled with fluid or semisolid substances, commonly found in many different areas of the body.

**CYTOKINES**
Cell signaling molecules that support cell-to-cell communication in immune responses and stimulate the movement of cells toward sites of inflammation, infection, and trauma.

**DETOXIFICATION**
A process of helping the body, especially the liver, to eliminate unwanted and potentially harmful substances.

**DIAMINE OXIDASE**
A digestive enzyme produced by the kidney, thymus, and gut lining, that helps break down excess histamine in the body.

**DIETARY FIBER**
A component of plant food that resists digestion because it cannot be broken down by human enzymes – also known as roughage.

**DIETITIAN**
An expert whose service is to provide food and nutrition information to prevent and treat disease.

**DIVERTICULITIS**
An inflammation or infection in one or more small pouches in the digestive tract.

**DYSBIOSIS**
A condition in which a persistent imbalance in the gut microbial community leads to health problems.

**ELECTROLYTES**
Minerals in the blood that help to regulate and control the balance of fluids in the body.

**ELIMINATION DIET**
Involves removing foods from the diet that are suspected of compromising health.

**ENDOCRINE SYSTEM**
The body's communication network, consisting of a collection of glands that produce hormones.

**ENEMA**
An application technique in which fluid is injected into the lower bowel for various purposes.

**ENTERIC NERVOUS SYSTEM**
Commonly referred to as the "second brain" because it is an autonomous part of the central nervous system; it independently controls the gastrointestinal tract, among other things.

**ENZYMES**
Molecules, mainly proteins, found in cells to regulate and speed up chemical reactions without being altered themselves.

**EPICUTANEOUS PATCH TEST**
A method used to identify specific substances that cause allergic reactions.

**EPITHELIAL CELLS**
A single layer of cells held together by the cell junctions, having direct contact with the basement membrane, which protects the inner part of the body from the invasion of unwanted microbes. Since it has no blood vessels, it is nourished by substances from the underlying connective tissue.

**FALSE NEGATIVE RESULT**
A test result that incorrectly indicates that a condition is not met.

**FAT-SOLUBLE VITAMINS**
Vitamins A, D, E and K do not dissolve in water but are absorbed with dietary fats and promote growth, reproduction, and general health.

**FATTY ACID**
A building block of fat in the body and the food we eat, and an important source of energy for humans and animals.

**FATTY LIVER DISEASE**
An alcoholic or non-alcoholic liver disease, in which fat cannot be broken down appropriately, leading to damage of the liver and serious health problems such as type 2 diabetes.

**FECAL MICROBIOME TRANSPLANTATION**
A technique to change the composition of the microbiome in a patient, by transplanting fecal material from a healthy human donor into the colon.

**FECAL OCCULT BLOOD TEST**
A laboratory test that investigates whether there is any hidden (occult) blood in a stool sample.

**FERRITIN**
A protein that stores and releases iron when it is needed to produce more red blood cells.

**FIBROMYALGIA**
A condition that causes widespread pain in the body, often accompanied by fatigue, impaired sleep and memory, and mood swings. There is no cure, but symptoms can be relieved.

**FOLIC ACID**
A man-made version of the vitamin folate, a water-soluble vitamin that is important for cell growth and function, also known as vitamin B9.

**FOOD ALLERGY**
A life-threatening reaction of the immune system to an otherwise harmless food.

**FOOD SENSITIVITY**
Describes a wide range of reactions to a particular food that are not caused by the immune system.

**FUNCTIONAL DIARRHEA**
Characterized by chronic and frequent loose stools that is not explained by structural or biochemical abnormalities.

**FUNCTIONAL MEDICINE**
Medical doctors who specialize in the interactions of the body's systems to find the cause and correct treatment for a disease.

**GASTRIC ACID**
A highly acidic digestive fluid that is produced by the stomach's lining to help digest food – also known as gastric juice or stomach acid.

**GASTROENTERITIS**
A common, usually short-term illness associated with infection and inflammation of the gastrointestinal tract.

**GASTROESOPHAGEAL REFLUX DISEASE**
A chronic digestive disorder in which acid from the stomach rises into the esophagus, causing burning and heartburn.

**GLIADIN PROTEIN**
A protein found in grains such as wheat that produces gluten, which is a causative for celiac disease.

**GLUTAMINE**
The most abundant amino acid in the body, which is produced by the body and can also be obtained from food.

**GLYCEMIC INDEX**
A method of ranking carbohydrate foods based on how quickly they are digested and increase blood sugar (glucose) levels.

**GOOD MANUFACTURING PRACTICES**
A system that complies with the guidelines and regulations recommended by the authorities to ensure the quality standards of the products manufactured.

**GRAM-NEGATIVE BACTERIA**
Strains of bacteria that can cause infections throughout the body and resist antibiotics due to their characteristic structure, making them a serious health problem in the world.

**GUT-BRAIN AXIS**
A bidirectional link between the central nervous system and the enteric nervous system.

**GUT FLORA**
See microbiome.

**HEIDELBERG STOMACH ACID TEST**
A method of diagnosing hypochlorhydria, that is, insufficient hydrochloric acid in the stomach, by swallowing a small radio transmitter capsule.

**HELICOBACTER PYLORI**
A bacteria in the digestive tract that attacks the stomach lining causing ulcers – a common reason for digestive disorders.

**HISTAMINE INTOLERANCE**
A condition in which there is an overproduction of histamine, or an inability to break it down, in the body.

**HOMEOSTASIS**
A biological system with self-regulating processes that seek to keep the body in a stable state at all levels and times to ensure survival.

**HORMONE**
A fat-based molecule produced by many organs in the body that is released directly into the bloodstream and distributed throughout the body to control a variety of functions.

**HYDROCHLORIC ACID**
A component of the dietary supplement betaine HCL, which increases the acidity of the stomach and thus supports digestion and helps eliminate bacteria and viruses in the stomach. Low levels of stomach acid impair the body's ability to digest and absorb nutrients.

## INFLAMMATION
The process by which the immune system defends the body against harmful pathogens, infections, injuries, and toxins to heal itself.

## INFLAMMATORY BOWEL DISEASE
Represents a group of intestinal disorders in which there is persistent inflammation in the gastrointestinal tract.

## IMMUNE SYSTEM
A complex network of biological processes that protects the body from disease.

## IMMUNOGLOBULINS (ANTIBODIES)
Proteins that are part of the immune system's defense strategy. If too few are in the blood, the likelihood of infection increases, while too many can be the cause of allergies or an overactive immune system.

## IMMUNOMODULATOR
A substance that can alter the immune response to a threat by stimulating or suppressing all or parts of the immune system.

## INNATE IMMUNE SYSTEM
The first defense strategy against pathogens, which can be physical, chemical, or cellular in nature.

## INSULIN
A hormone produced in the pancreas that regulates the metabolism of carbohydrates, fat, and protein.

## INTEGRATIVE MEDICINE
A branch of allopathic medicine that seeks to understand the overall well-being of the individual and does not focus on one condition. Doctors may use various forms of therapies and emphasize lifestyle changes.

## INTESTINAL PERMEABILITY
Indicates how permeable the intestinal barrier is. If the tight connection of the epithelial cells becomes too loose, substances that normally do not enter the blood can do so. Also known as leaky gut.

## JARISCH-HERXHEIMER REACTION
A reaction due to endotoxin substances released by the death of microorganisms during antimicrobial treatment or elimination diets, also known as "die-off" symptoms.

## KETONE BODIES
Water-soluble molecules produced by the liver during calorie restriction or strenuous exercise, to serve as an additional energy source.

## LACTO-FERMENTATION
A food preservation process that uses salt, water, and vegetables. During this process, bacteria break down the sugar in the food and form a lactic acid, giving the product a distinctive taste.

## LACTOBACILLI BACTERIA
A member of the lactic acidic, non-spore-forming bacteria that is part of the lacto-fermentation process and an integral part of the microbiome as it breaks down dietary fiber.

## LAUGHTER YOGA
A practice of breathing exercises and voluntary laughter, to reduce stress and enhance health and well-being.

## LUPUS
An autoimmune disease caused by the immune system that attacks the person's own tissues and can affect organs, joints, skin, and blood vessels.

## LYMPHOCYTE
A type of white blood cell that is part of the immune system and is found in the lymph.

## LYMPH
A clear to white fluid that flows through the lymphatic system and consists of lymphocytes and protein- and fat-containing fluid from the intestines.

## MALABSORPTION
A condition which occurs when the small intestine is unable to extract and absorb nutrients from food during the digestive process.

## MALNOURISHMENT/ MALNUTRITION
A condition in which the body does not receive enough nutrients, due to poor diet, lack of food, or because it is unable to metabolize foods.

## MEDITATION
Meditation is a technique for quieting the mind and achieving a state of consciousness that is different from the normal waking state.

## MEDULLA
A long stem-like structure located at the base of the brain, where it connects to the spinal cord. It helps transmit messages between these two parts of the body and regulates the cardiovascular and respiratory systems.

**MELATONIN**
A hormone that plays a role in the sleep-wake cycle and is released at night by the pineal gland.

**MERCURY**
A heavy metal that is toxic to humans and found in the environment, thus in food.

**METABOLISM**
A complex chemical process by which the body converts food and other substances into energy to perform daily functions.

**METABOLITES**
Small molecules produced during metabolism.

**MICROBIOTA**
The collective of microorganisms such as bacteria, archaea, fungi and other single-celled organisms in a given environment, for example in the gut or on the skin.

**MICROBIOME**
Refers to the totality of the genomes of microorganisms in a given environment, including all their genetic material such as DNA and RNA.

**MICROORGANISM**
Microscopic organisms, including single-celled organisms or a colony of cells.

**MICROSCOPIC COLITIS**
A disease in which the colon is inflamed. The tissue of the colon must be examined under a microscope to identify it.

**MICROVILLI**
A microscopic finger-like projection found on the surface of larger cells.

**MOTILITY**
The coordination of movement in the gastrointestinal tract required to digest food.

**MUCOSA**
A thick, moist, membrane that lines certain parts of the inside of the body.

**NEUROTOXIN**
Toxins that alter the tissues and functions of the nervous system.

**NEUROTRANSMITTER**
Chemical messengers that transmit signals through synapses from one neuron to another neuron, a muscle, or a gland.

**NUTRITIONIST**
An expert in the field of food and nutrients who takes a scientific approach and establishes or implements programs for clients to improve their nutritional intake.

**OSMOSIS**
The movement of water molecules from a place of low solute concentration to a place of high solute concentration to maintain balance.

**PANTOTHENIC ACID**
A water-soluble vitamin, B5. Also known as pantothenate.

**PARASITE INFECTION**
A parasite is an organism that lives in or on a host, such as a human or animal. A parasitic infection can cause harm by affecting the host's organ system.

**PEPSIN**
An abundant protein digestive enzyme that chemically breaks down proteins into shorter chains of amino acids.

**PEPTIDES**
A class of organic compounds that consist of various numbers of amino acids, typically 2-50 amino acids, that are linked by peptide bonds.

**PERIPHERAL NERVOUS SYSTEM**
One of two components of the nervous system, encompassing the nerves outside the brain and spinal cord.

**PERISTALSIS**
Wave-like muscle contractions that move food through the digestive tract.

**PH LEVEL**
A scale used in chemistry to indicate the acidity or basicity of water-based solutions such as gastric fluid.

**PIGMENT BILIRUBIN**
A yellow-brownish pigment of bile secreted by the liver that gives feces its characteristic color. Too much bilirubin can cause yellowing of the skin and eyes (jaundice).

**PLASMA**
The largest component of blood; a clear to yellowish aqueous substance that holds blood cells, protein, and other components in suspension.

**POLYMERASE CHAIN REACTION TEST**
A method of amplifying small sections of DNA used, for example, to identify genetic relationships, for cloning, or to detect pathogens.

**POST-INFECTIOUS IRRITABLE BOWEL SYNDROME**
A condition that can occur after acute gastroenteritis and creates symptoms of IBS.

**PROGESTERONE CREAM**
A hormone replacement therapy designed to help relieve the symptoms of menopause.

**PRO-INFLAMMATORY**
Promotes or stimulates inflammation

**PROKINETIC AGENT**
An agent, pharmaceutical or herbal, that increases gastrointestinal motility by increasing contractions but does not affect the rhythm.

**PROLAMIN**
A plant storage protein found mainly in seeds high in proline amino acid, such as wheat, barley, rye, corn, sorghum, and oats

**PSEUDO-ALLERGIES**
A reaction that mimics the signs of a true allergy but is not associated with the immune system.

**PSYCHOSOMATIC DISORDERS**
Physical symptoms that are caused or influenced by mental factors, such as internal conflict or stress.

**RIFAXIMIN (US: XIFAXAN, CANADA: ZAXINE)**
A semi-synthetic, non-systemic oral rifamycin-based antibiotic that does not pass through the gastrointestinal wall into the bloodstream. Commonly used for traveler's diarrhea and IBS because it stops the growth of bacteria that cause diarrhea.

**RESTLESS LEGS (WILLIS-EKBORN DISEASE)**
A neurological disorder characterized by the urge to move the legs when sitting or lying down, which can lead to sleep disturbances.

**ROME IV CRITERIA**
A method for diagnosing IBS released by the Rome Foundation.

**RUBBER BAND LIGATION**
A non-surgical treatment in which hemorrhoids are tied off at their base with a rubber band to stop the flow of blood, which usually causes them to shrink and fall off (along with the band).

**SEROTONIN**
A chemical that transmits messages between nerve cells and acts in various functions in the body – also known as the "happy hormone".

**SHORT-CHAIN FATTY ACIDS**
Metabolites produced in the intestinal microbiota during fermentation of dietary fiber.

**STEATORRHEA**
Excess fat in the stool and a clinical characteristic of fat malabsorption that occurs in conditions such as celiac disease and exocrine pancreatic insufficiency.

**T-CELLS**
White blood cells, which are part of the immune system, that focus on attacking specific foreign particles, cells, and viruses.

**TELOMERES**
A distinctive structure with specialized proteins located at both ends of each chromosome, and an essential part of human cells.

**THIRD-PARTY LABORATORY ANALYSIS**
An independent testing laboratory that performs scientific tests to analyze a product.

**TOTAL CHOLESTEROL**
A measure of the total amount of cholesterol in the blood including high-density lipoprotein and low-density lipoprotein.

**TRADITIONAL CHINESE MEDICINE**
Complementary therapy referring to ancient Chinese practices that seek to establish balance in the body and promote life forces (also called qi).

**TREATMENT PROTOCOL**
A written direction for the treatment of a disease or condition.

**ULCERATIVE COLITIS**
An inflammatory bowel disease that causes irritation, inflammation, and ulcers in the colon.

**VILLUS (PL VILLI)**
A small finger-like projection that extends into the lumen of the small intestine and increases the surface area for food absorption.

**VIPASSANA MEDITATION**
A Buddhist insight meditation usually practiced over ten days in silence.

**VISCERAL HYPERSENSITIVITY**
A phenomenon in which pain and discomfort is experienced in the soft internal organs (visceral organs) such as the lungs, heart, and organs of the digestive tract.

# RESOURCES

## BOOKS

*Accessing The Healing Power of The Vagus Nerve. Self-Help Exercises for Anxiety, Depression, Trauma, And Autism.* Stanley Rosenberg, Kindle edition, 2017, North Atlantic Books, California. ISBN 978-1-62317-025-7 (Kindle edition)

*Activate Your Vagus Nerve. Unleash Your Body's Natural Ability to Heal.* Dr. Navaz Habib, 2019, Ulysses Press, US. ISBN 978-1-61243-910-5 (Kindle edition)

*A Step-By-Step Guide to Stop Bloating & Heal Your Gut. Clean low* FODMAP *Diet. 101 Clean, unprocessed, super healthy Mediterranean-Inspired, Gluten-Free Recipes, Dietitian-Approved.* Aliki Economides and Irini Hadjisavva, 2021, Livani Publishing Organization S.A. ISBN 978-960-3542-8 (PB)

*Ayurvedic Medicine. The Principles of Traditional Practice.* Sebastian Pole, 2013, Singing Dragon, London and Philadelphia. ISBN 978-1-84819-113-6 (HC)

*Breath. The New Science of a Lost Art.* James Nestor, 2020, Penguin Random House, UK. ISBN 978-0-241-28908-2 (PB)

*Breaking the Vicious Cycle. Intestinal Health Through Diet.* Elaine Gloria Gottschall, 1994, Kirkton Press. ISBN: 0969276818 (PB)

*Digestive Health with Real Food. A practical guide to an anti-inflammatory, low-irritant, nutrient-dense diet for IBS & other digestive issues.* Aglaée Jacob, 2013, Paleo Media Group, Oregon. ISBN 13: 978-0-9887172-0-6 (Kindle edition)

*Emotional Inflammation. Discover Your Triggers and Reclaim Your Equilibrium During Anxious Times.* Lise Van Susteren, MD and Stacey Colino, 2020, Sounds True. ISBN 9781683644569 (Kindle edition)

*Fast Tract Digestion, IBS. A Revolutionary Diet Approach to Treat and Prevent Irritable Bowel Syndrome.* Norman Robillard, PhD, 2013, Self Health Publishing, Massachusetts. ISBN 978-0-9766425-2-7 (Kindle edition)

*Fiber Fueled. The Plant-Based Gut Health Program for Losing Weight, Restoring Health, and Optimizing Your Microbiome.* Will Bulsiewicz, 2020, Avery - an imprint of Penguin Random House, New York. ISBN 978059084571 (Kindle edition)

*Healthy Gut, Healthy You. The Personalized Plan to Transform Your Health from the Inside Out.* Dr. Michael Ruscio, 2018, The Ruscio Institute, LLC, Las Vegas. ISBN 978-0-99976-681-1 (Kindle edition)

*Miracles through Pranic Healing. Practical Manual on Energy Healing.* Master Choa Kok Sui, 2004, Fourth edition, Institute for Inner Studies Publishing Foundation, Philippines. ISBN 971-0376-04-7 (PB)

*Take Control of Your IBS. The complete guide to manage your symptoms.* Professor Peter Whorwell, 2017, Vermilion, an imprint of Ebury Publishing, London. Penguin Random House, UK. ISBN 9781473528758 (Kindle edition)

The Activated Grain Method. Easy, Nutritious and Delicious Gluten Free Recipes using The Active Grain Method. Todd Stream Cameron, 2016. https://activatedgrainmethod.com.au (PB)

*The Anti-Anxiety Food Solution. How the Food You Eat Can Help You Calm Your Anxious Mind, Improve Your Mood and End Cravings.* Trudy Scott, CN, 2011, Viking

Penguin a division of Penguin Group, USA. ISBN 978-1-57224-925-7 (PB)

*The Clever Guts Diet. How to Revolutionise Your Body from the Inside Out.* Dr. Michael Mosley, 2017, Short books, London. ISBN 978-1-78072-304-4 (PB)

*The Fast Diet. Lose weight, stay healthy, live longer.* Dr. Michael Mosley and Mimi Spencer, 2013, Short books, London. ISBN 978-1-78072-237-5. (PB)

*The Happy Kitchen. Good Mood Food.* Rachel Kelly with Alice Mackintosh, 2017, Short Books, London. ISBN 978-1-78072-296-2 (PB)

*The Longevity Diet. Discover the New Science to Slow Aging, Fight Disease and Manage Your Weight.* Dr. Valter Longo, 2018, Penguin Random House, Australia. ISBN 9780143788379 (PB)

*The Paleo Approach. Reverse Autoimmune Disease and Heal Your Body.* Sarah Ballantyne, PhD, 2013, Victory Belt Publishing, Las Vegas. ISBN 13: 978-1-936608-39-3 (PB)

*The Pocket Guide to The Polyvagal Theory. The Transformative Power of Feeling Safe.* Stephen W. Porges, 2017, W.W. Norton & Company, New York. ISBN 978-0-393-70853-0 (Kindle edition)

*The Slow Down Diet. Eating for Pleasure, Energy and Weight Loss. An 8-Week Breakthrough Program.* Marc David, 2015, Healing Arts Press. ISBN 978-1-62055-509-5 (Kindle edition)

*Your Hands can Heal.* Stephen Co, Eric B. Robins and John Merryman, 2002, Atria, New York. ISBN 978-0-7432-4305-6 (PB)

## OTHER RESOURCES

Aggregate Nutrient Density Index: https://www.drfuhrman.com/blog/128/andi-food-scores-rating-the-nutrient-density-of-foods

America Academy of Allergy Asthma & Immunology: https://www.aaaai.org

American Gut and British Gut Project: https://microsetta.ucsd.edu

Australian Government (low mercery fish): https://www.foodauthority.nsw.gov.au

Autoimmune association (Disease list): https://autoimmune.org/disease-information

Brain.fm: https://www.brain.fm

Coeliac Australia: https://www.coeliac.org.au

Core Energetics: https://www.coreenergetics.org

Eat Forum: https://eatforum.org

Elemental diet (homemade version): https://www.siboinfo.com/elemental-formula.html

Emotional Freedom Technique: https://www.emofree.com

Environmental Working Group: https://www.ewg.org/foodnews/dirty-dozen.php

f.lux: https://justgetflux.com

Food intolerance network and FAILSAFE: https://www.fedup.com.au

Food freedom with Ayurveda: https://www.muditainstitute.com/courses

FoodPrint: https://foodprint.org

Gottschall, Elaine: http://www.breakingtheviciouscycle.info

Healthy Eating Plate, Harvard T.H. Chan: https://www.hsph.harvard.edu/nutritionsource/healthy-eating-plate

HeartMath Institute: https://www.heartmath.org

Ileocecal valve maneuver: https://www.youtube.com/watch?v=ATmSVdeSo_U

Mosley, Michael. The fast 800 dietary program: https://thefast800.com

National Institute of Environmental Health Sciences: https://www.niehs.nih.gov

NSW Food Authority: https://www.foodauthority.nsw.gov.au

Nutrient dense foods list: Kim, S., et. al. 2015. "Uncovering the Nutritional Landscape of Food". https://doi.org/10.1371/journal.pone.0118697

Redshift: http://jonls.dk/redshift

Royal Melbourne Hospital, free service for mental health (formally IBS Clinic): https://www.ibs.mindovergut.com

Seasonal Food Guide Australia: http://seasonalfoodguide.com

SIBO Bi-Phasic Diet: https://www.thesibodoctor.com/sibo-bi-phasic-diet-free-downloads

SIBO SOS, Shivan Sarna: https://sibosos.com

SIBO Specific Food Guide: https://www.siboinfo.com/diet.html

Siebecker, Allison: https://www.siboinfo.com

Sleep Health Foundation: https://www.sleephealthfoundation.org.au

Smiling Mind: https://www.smilingmind.com.au

The Australian Government of NSW Food Authority: https://www.foodauthority.nsw.gov.au

The Fast Tract Diet calculator: https://digestivehealthinstitute.org/fp-calculator

The Institute for Inner Studies: https://www.globalpranichealing.com

The low-FODMAP Diet, Monash University: https://www.monashfodmap.com

The National Sleep Foundation: https://www.sleepfoundation.org

Thich Nhat Hanh: https://plumvillage.org

United States Department of Agriculture: https://www.nal.usda.gov/fnic (food database) and https://fdc.nal.usda.gov (general nutrition Information)

Weil, Andrew. Breathing exercise: https://www.drweil.com/videos-features/videos/breathing-exercises-4-7-8-breath

World Helpline: http://worldhelplines.org

# REFERENCES

## QUOTE

Bischoff, S. 2011. "'Gut health': a new objective in medicine?" *BMC Medicine* 9 (24). https://doi.org/10.1186/1741-7015-9-24

## IRRITABLE BOWEL SYNDROME

Agrawal, A., et. al. 2008. "Bloating and Distention in Irritable Bowel Syndrome: The Role of Visceral Sensation". *Gastroenterology* 134 (7): 1882-1889. https://doi.org/10.1053/j.gastro.2008.02.096

Arzani, M., et. al., 2020. "Gut-brain Axis and migraine headache: a comprehensive review". *The Journal of Headache and Pain* 21 (1). https://doi.org/10.1186/s10194-020-1078-9

Azpiroz, F., et. al. 2007. "Mechanisms of hypersensitivity in IBS and functional disorders". *Neurogastroenterology & Motility* 19 (s1): 62-88. https://doi.org/10.1111/j.1365-2982.2006.00875.x

Berres, I. 2018. "Iberogast: Streit um Nebenwirkungen des Magen-Darm-Mittels". https://www.spiegel.de/gesundheit/diagnose/iberogast-streit-um-nebenwirkungen-des-magen-darm-mittelsa-1195411.html

Bruta, K., et. al. 2021. "The role of Serotonin and Diet in the prevalence of Irritable Bowel Syndrome: a Systematic Review". *Translational Medicine Communications* 6 (1). https://doi.org/10.1186/s41231-020-00081-y

Dumitrașcu, D. L., et. al. 2007. "Therapy of the Postinfectious Irritable Bowel Syndrome: An Update". Medicine and Pharmacy Reports 90 (2): 133-138. https://doi.org/10.15386/cjmed-752

Dwyer, E. 2019. "Gut Dysbiosis". Monash University Australia, FODMAP blog. http://www.monashfodmap.com/blog/gut-dysbiosis

Gemelli Biotech. n.d. "There's Now a Way to Diagnose IBS With a Simple Blood Test". https://www.ibssmart.com

Ghoshal, U. C., et. al. 2017. "Small Intestinal Bacterial Overgrowth and Irritable Bowel Syndrome: A Bridge between Functional Organic Dichotomy". *Gut and Liver* 11 (2): 196-208. https://doi.org/10.5009/gnl16126

GI Society. n.d. "Irritable Bowel Syndrome (IBS) and Serotonin". https://badgut.org/information-centre/a-z-digestive-topics/ibs-and-serotonin

Iacob, T., et. al. 2007. "Therapy of the Postinfectious Irritable Bowel Syndrome: An Update". *Medicine and Pharmacy Reports* 90 (2): 133-138. https://doi.org/10.15386/cjmed-752

IBS Clinic. "What is IBS Clinic?". https://www.ibs.mindovergut.com

John Hopkins Medicine. n.d. "Irritable Bowel Syndrome (IBS): Introduction". [PDF]. John Hopkins Medicine Health Library. https://www.hopkinsmedicine.org/gastroenterology_hepatology/_pdfs/small_large_intestine/irritable_bowel_byndrome_IBS.pdf

Kim, Y. S., et. al. 2018. "Sex-Gender Differences in Irritable Bowel Syndrome". *Journal of Neurogastroenterology and Motility* 24 (4): 544-558. https://doi.org/10.5056/jnm18082

Lacy, B., et. al. 2017. "Rome Criteria and a Diagnostic Approach to Irritable Bowel Syndrome". *Journal of Clinical Medicine* 6 (11). https://doi.org/10.3390/jcm6110099

McIntosh, J. 2015. "IBS can be quickly diagnosed with new blood test". https://www.medicalnewstoday.com/articles/294195

MedlinePlus. n.d. "Rifaximin". https://medlineplus.gov/druginfo/meds/a604027.html

Menees, S., et. al. 2018. "The gut microbiome and Irritable Bowel Syndrome". *F1000Research* 7. https://doi.org/10.12688/f1000research.14592.1

Mitchell, H., et. al. 2019. "Review article: implementation of a diet low in FODMAPs for patients with Irritable Bowel Syndrome-directions for future research". *Alimentary Pharmacology & Therapeutics* 49 (2): 124-139. https://doi.org/10.1111/apt.15079

Muir, J., et. al. 2016. "Diet for gastro: the low FODMAP diet during the recovery phase after gastroenteritis". Monash University Australia, FODMAP blog. http://www.monashfodmap.com/blog/diet-for-gastro-low-fodmap-diet-during

Peters, S. 2019. "How hypnotherapy is helping treat Irritable Bowel Syndrome (IBS) sufferers". Monash University Australia. https://lens.monash.edu/@mecine-health/2019/06/24/1351605/how-hypnotherapy-is-helping-people-suffering-from-irritable-bowel-syndrome-ibs

Pimentel, M. 2017. "Irritable Bowel Syndrome with Dr. Mark Pimentel". Interview by Ben Weitz. *YouTube: Ben Weitz.* [Embedded Video]. https://www.youtube.com/watch?v=ARaEnKQIPTo

Rezaie, A., and Cedars-Sinai Medical Center. 2018. "Efficacy and Safety of SYN-010 in IBS-C". U.S. National Library of Medicine. https://clinicaltrials.gov/ct2/show/NCT03763175

Rodiño-Janeiro, B. K., et. al. 2018. "A Review of Microbiota and Irritable Bowel Syndrome: Future in Therapies". *Advances in Therapy* 35 (3): 289-310. https://doi.org/10.1007/s12325-018-0673-5

Sansone, R. A., et. al. 2015. "Irritable Bowel Syndrome: Relationships with abuse in childhood". *Innov Clin Neurosci* 12 (5-6): 34-7. https://www.ncbi.nlm.nih.gov/pubmed/26155376

Siebecker, A. 2013. "Small Intestine Bacterial Overgrowth: Often ignored cause of Irritable Bowel Syndrome". https://www.townsendletter.com/FebMarch2013/ibs0213.html

Sibotest. n.d. "IBS-smart™ now available in Australia". https://sibotest.com/pages/get_IBS-smart

Synthetic Biologics. 2020. "Synthetic Biologics Provides Update on Investigator-Sponsored Phase 2b Clinical Study of SYN-010 in IBS-C Patients". Cision PR Newswire. https://www.prnewswire.com/news-releases/synthetic-biologics-provides-update-on-investigator-sponsored-phase-2b-clinical-study-of-syn-010-in-ibs-c-patients-301144645.html

Vahora, I. S., et. al. 2020. "How Serotonin Level Fluctuation Affects the Effectiveness of Treatment in Irritable Bowel Syndrome". *Cureus*. https://doi.org/10.7759/cureus.9871

Whorwell, Peter. 2017. *Take Control of Your IBS. The complete guide to manage your symptoms*. Vermilion, an imprint of Ebury Publishing, London. Penguin Random House. [Kindle] ISBN 9781473528758

## SMALL INTESTINAL BACTERIAL OVERGROWTH

Bischoff, S. C. 2011. "'Gut health': A new objective in medicine?" *BMC Medicine* 9 (24). https://bmcmedicine.biomedcentral.com/articles/10.1186/1741-7015-9-24

Bures, J., et. al. 2010. "Small Intestinal Bacterial Overgrowth Syndrome." World J Gastroenterol 16 (24): 2978-90. https://doi.org/10.3748/wjg.v16.i24.2978

Dukowicz, A. C., et. al. 2007. "Small intestinal bacterial overgrowth: a comprehensive review." *Gastroenterol Hepatol (N Y)* 3 (2): 112-22. https://www.ncbi.nlm.nih.gov/pubmed/21960820

Ghoshal, U. C., et. al. 2017. "Small Intestinal Bacterial Overgrowth and Irritable Bowel Syndrome: A Bridge between Functional Organic Dichotomy." *Gut and Liver* 11 (2): 196-208. https://doi.org/10.5009/gnl16126

Kresser, C. 2015. "4 Little-Known Causes of Restless Legs Syndrome Restless Legs Syndrome". https://chriskresser.com/4-little-known-causes-of-restless-legs-syndrome

Marchesi, J. R., et. al. 2015. "The vocabulary of microbiome research: a proposal." Microbiome 3: 31. https://doi.org/10.1186/s40168-015-0094-5

Pimentel, M., et. al. 2020. "ACG clinical guideline: Small Intestinal Bacterial Overgrowth." *The American Journal of Gastroenterology* 115 (2): 165-178. https://doi.org/10.14309/ajg.0000000000000501

Mayo Clinic staff. "Diverticulitis." Mayo Foundation. https://www.mayoclinic.org/diseases-conditions/diverticulitis/symptoms-causes/syc-20371758

Sachdev, A. H., et. al. 2013. "Gastrointestinal bacterial overgrowth: pathogenesis and clinical significance." *Therapeutic Advances in Chronic Disease* 4 (5): 223-231. https://doi.org/10.1177/2040622313496126

Siebecker, A. n.d. "Associated Diseases." SIBO-Small Intestinal Bacterial Overgrowth. https://www.siboinfo.com/associated-diseases.html

Takakura, W., et. al. 2020. "Small Intestinal Bacterial Overgrowth and Irritable Bowel Syndrome – An Update." *Frontiers in Psychiatry* 11. https://doi.org/10.3389/fpsyt.2020.00664

Thomas, L. 2019. "Fibromyalgia and Small Intestinal Bacterial Overgrowth (SIBO)." https://www.news-medical.net/health/Fibromyalgia-and-Small-Intestinal-Bacterial-Overgrowth-(SIBO).aspx

Tuddenham, S., et. al. 2015. "The intestinal microbiome and health." *Current Opinion in Infectious Diseases* 28 (5): 464-470. https://doi.org/10.1097/qco.0000000000000196

Weinstock, L. B., et. al. 2008. "Restless legs syndrome in patients with Irritable Bowel Syndrome: Response to Small Intestinal Bacterial Overgrowth Therapy." *Dig Dis Sci* 53 (5): 1252-6. https://doi.org/10.1007/s10620-007-0021-0

## HOW DO I KNOW THAT I HAVE SIBO?

Kresser, C. 2015. "4 Little-Known Causes of Restless Legs Syndrome Restless Legs Syndrome".https://chriskresser.com/4-little-known-causes-of-restless-legs-syndrome

Mayo Clinic. n.d. "Capsule endoscopy". https://www.mayoclinic.org/tests-procedures/capsule-endoscopy/about/pac-20393366

Siebecker, A. n.d. "Associated Diseases". SIBO-Small intestinal Bacterial Overgrowth. https://www.siboinfo.com/associated-diseases.html

Siebecker, A., et. al. 2013. "Small Intestine Bacterial Overgrowth: Often ignored cause of Irritable Bowel Syndrome". https://www.townsendletter.com/FebMarch2013/ibs0213.html

## HYDROGEN BREATH TEST

Jacobi, N. n.d. "Breath Testing for SIBO with Dr Nirala Jacobi," Interview by Carly Woods. *The SIBO Doctor Podcast, Ep 7*. [Audio]. https://www.thesibodoctor.com/2017/03/14/the-sibo-doctor-podcast-dr-nirala-jacobi-breath-testing-for-sibo

Pandit, A. 2020. "Gemelli Biotech Launches Novel Breath Test Measuring Hydrogen, Methane and Hydrogen Sulfide". Businesswire. https://www.businesswire.com/news/home/20201027005024/en/Gemelli-Biotech-Launches-Novel-Breath-Test-Measuring-Hydrogen-Methane-and-Hydrogen-Sulfide

Siebecker, A. 2018. "IBS and SIBO foundations & fundamentals". Interview by Shivan Sarna. *IBS and SIBO SOS summit*. [Transcript]. Chronic Condition Rescue. https://sibosos.com/summits

Swain, P., et. al. 2004. "Role of video endoscopy in managing small bowel disease". *Gut* 53 (12): 1866-1875. https://doi.org/10.1136/gut.2003.035576

## HYDROGEN VS. METHANE

Takakura, W., et. al. 2020. "Small Intestinal Bacterial Overgrowth and Irritable Bowel Syndrome – An Update". *Frontiers in Psychiatry* 11. https://doi.org/10.3389/fpsyt.2020.00664

## ARCHAEA

Gaci, N., et. al. 2014. "Archaea and the human gut: New beginning of an old story". World Journal of Gastroenterology 20 (43). https://doi.org/10.3748/wjg.v20.i43.16062

Hogan, M. C. 2012. "Archaea". Encyclopedia of Life. https://eol.org/docs/discover/archaea

Lee, H.-S. 2013. "Diversity of Halophilic Archaea in Fermented Foods and Human Intestines and Their Application". *Journal of Microbiology and Biotechnology* 23 (12): 1645-1653. https://doi.org/10.4014/jmb.1308.08015

Wolf, J. 2017. "New Insight into Archaeal Members of the Human Microbiome". American Society for Microbiology. https://www.asm.org/Articles/2017/November/mBiosphere-(48)

## HYDROGEN DOMINANT SIBO (D)

Sachdev, A. H., et. al. 2013. "Gastrointestinal bacterial overgrowth: pathogenesis and clinical significance". *Therapeutic Advances in Chronic Disease* 4 (5): 223-231. https://doi.org/10.1177/2040622313496126

## INTESTINAL METHANOGEN OVERGROWTH

Mather, R., et. al. 2013. "Methane and Hydrogen Positivity on Breath Test Is Associated With Greater Body Mass Index and Body Fat". *The Journal of Clinical Endocrinology & Metabolism* 98 (4): E698-E702. https://doi.org/10.1210/jc.2012-3144

Mather, R., et. al. 2013. "Intestinal Methanobrevibacter smithii but not total bacteria is related to diet-induced weight gain in rats". *Wiley Online Library, Obesity* 21 (4): 748-754. https://doi.org/10.1002/oby.20277

Peled, Y., et. al. 1985. "The Development of Methane Production in Childhood and Adolescence". *Journal of Pediatric Gastroenterology and Nutrition* 4 (4): 575-579. https://journals.lww.com/jpgn/Abstract/1985/08000/The_Development_of_Methane_Production_in_Childhood.13.aspx

Triantafyllou, K., et. al. 2014. "Methanogens, Methane and Gastrointestinal Motility". *Journal of Neuro-gastroenterology and Motility* 20 (1): 31-40. https://doi.org/10.5056/jnm.2014.20.1.31

## HYDROGEN DOMINANT SIBO (D)

Sachdev, A. H., et. al. 2013. "Gastrointestinal bacterial overgrowth: pathogenesis and clinical significance". *Therapeutic Advances in Chronic Disease* 4 (5): 223-231. https://doi.org/10.1177/2040622313496126

## HYDROGEN SULFIDE

Businesswire, 2020. "Gemelli Biotech Launches Novel Breath Test Measuring Hydrogen, Methane and Hydrogen Sulfide". https://www.businesswire.com/news/home/20201027005024/en/Gemelli-Biotech-Launches-Novel-Breath-Test-Measuring-Hydrogen-Methane-and-Hydrogen-Sulfide

Takakura, W., et. al. 2020. "Sa1215 Using a Novel 4-Gas Breath Test Device, Multivariable Analysis Reveals an Association between Excessive Hydrogen Sulfide on Breath Testing and Heartburn". *Gastroenterology, AGA Abstracts* 158 (6). https://doi.org/10.1016/S0016-5085(20)31487-6

Trio smart. n.d. "Get a more complete picture". https://www.triosmartbreath.com

## SULFUR, SULFATE, SULFITE

Canani, R. B. 2011. "Potential beneficial effects of butyrate in intestinal and extraintestinal diseases". *World Journal of Gastroenterology* 17 (12). https://doi.org/10.3748/wjg.v17.i12.1519

Jacobi, N., 2018. "2018 SIBO Highlights with Dr Nirala Jacobi". *The SIBO Doctor Podcast, Ep 34.* [Audio]. https://www.thesibodoctor.com/2018/12/24/2018-sibo-highlights-nirala-jacobi/?v=6c-c98ba2045f

Miller, C. A. 2018. "Difference Between Sulfide and Sulfite". Atomic & Molecular Structure. https://sciencing.com/difference-between-sulfide-sulfite-8559544.html

Nigh, G. 2017. "Sulfur Metabolism demystified and an alternative view of SIBO". Interview by Shivan Sarna. *SIBO SOS Summit 2017.* [Transcript]. Chronic Condition Rescue. https://sibosos.com/summits

Nigh, G. 2018. "Hydrogen Sulfide SIBO with Dr. Nigh". Interview by Josh Sullivan. *YouTube: SIBO Survivor.* [Embedded Video]. https://www.youtube.com/watch?v=jbBiOaSd4iU

Yarnell, E. 2010. "Sulfur-Rich foods and Ulcerative Colitis". [PDF]. http://citeseerx.ist.psu.edu/viewdoc/download?doi=10.1.1.693.6424&rep=rep1&type=pdf

Yarnell, E. n.d. "SIBO, IBS and Herbal Medicine with Dr Eric Yarnell," Interview by Nirala Jacobi. *The SIBO Doctor Podcast, Ep 24.* [Audio]. https://www.thesibodoctor.com/2018/04/28/sibo-ibs-herbal-medicine-dr-eric-yarnell/?v=6cc98ba2045f

## SMALL INTESTINAL FUNGAL OVERGROWTH

Encyclopedia. 2018. "Fungal infections". https://www.encyclopedia.com/medicne/diseases-and-conditions/pathology/fungal-infections

Erdogan, A., et. al. 2015. "Small intestinal fungal overgrowth". *Current Gastroenterology Reports* 17 (4):16. https://doi.org/10.1007/s11894-015-0436-2

Hamaza, A., et. al. 2015. "Small Intestinal Bacterial Overgrowth (SIBO) and Fungal Overgrowth (SIFO): A Frequent and Unrecognized Complication of Colectomy: ACG Category Award: Presidential Poster 2396". *American Journal of Gastroenterology* 110: S995. https://doi.org/10.14309/00000434-201510001-02397

Hogg, M. 2018. "Candida & Gut Dysbiosis". The Environmental Illness Resource. https://www.ei-resource.org/illness-information/environmental-illnesses/candida-and-gut-dysbiosis

Jacobs, C., et. al. 2013. "Dysmotility and proton pump inhibitor use are independent risk factors for small intestinal bacterial and/or fungal overgrowth".

*Alimentary Pharmacology & Therapeutics* 37 (11): 1103-1111. https://doi.org/10.1111/apt.12304

Kumar, P., et. al. 2017. "Aflatoxins: A Global Concern for Food Safety, Human Health and Their Management". *Frontiers in Microbiology* 07. https://doi.org/10.3389/fmicb.2016.02170

Lyz, X., et . al. 2016. "Efficacy of nystatin for the treatment of oral candidiasis: a systematic review and meta-analysis". *Drug Design, Development and Therapy* 10: 1161-1171. https://doi.org/10.2147/DDDT.S100795

Ruscio, M. 2019. "Everything You Need to Know about SIFO (Small Intestinal Fungal Overgrowth)". https://drruscio.com/everything-need-know-sifo-small-intestinal-fungal-overgrowth

Sheweita, S. A., et.al. Li. 2017. "Reduction of Aflatoxin B1 Toxicity by Lactobacillus plantarum C88: A Potential Probiotic Strain Isolated from Chinese Traditional Fermented Food "Tofu"". *Plos One* 12 (1). https://doi.org/10.1371/journal.pone.0170109

The Great Plains Laboratory. n.d. "Organic Acids Test". https://www.greatplainslaboratory.com/organic-acids-test

World Health Organization. 2009. *WHO guidelines for indoor air quality: Dampness and mould.* WHO Regional Office for Europe. https://apps.who.int/iris/handle/10665/164348

World Health Organization. 2018. "Mycotoxins". https://www.who.int/news-room/fact-sheets/detail/mycotoxins

## SIBO TREATMENT (STAGE 1-3)

Achufusi, T. G. O., et. al. 2020. "Small Intestinal Bacterial Overgrowth: Comprehensive Review of Diagnosis, Prevention, and Treatment Methods". *Cureus* 12 (6): e8860. https://doi.org/10.7759/cureus.8860

Ghoshal, U. C., et.al. 2017. "Small Intestinal Bacterial Overgrowth and Irritable Bowel Syndrome: A Bridge between Functional Organic Dichotomy". *Gut and Liver* 11 (2): 196-208. https://doi.org/10.5009/gnl16126

Jacobi, N. 2016. "The SIBO Bi-Phasic Diet, testing and herbal treatments with Dr. Nirala Jacobi". Interview by Rebecca Coomes. *The Healthy Gut Podcast, Ep. 4.* [Audio]. https://www.thehealthygut.com/podcast/herbaltreatments

Lindemann, B. 2019. "Pathogen & Parasite Die-off Symptoms: How to manage Detox Side-Effects". The functional gut health clinic. https://bellalindemann.com/blog/pathogen-parasite-die-off-symptoms

National Center for Complementary and Integrative Health. 2019. "Probiotics: What you need to know". National Institutes of Health. https://www.nccih.nih.gov/health/probiotics-what-you-need-to-know

Ruscio, M. 2020. "SIBO, Probiotics, and Your Gut Health: A Long-Term Strategy". https://drruscio.com/sibo-probiotics

Sorathia, S. J., et. al. 2021. "Small Intestinal Bacterial Overgrowth". NCBI Bookshelf. StatPearls Publishing. https://pubmed.ncbi.nlm.nih.gov/31536241

## ANTIMICROBIALS

Boltin, D., et. al. 2014. "Rifaximin for Small Intestinal Bacterial Overgrowth in patients without Irritable Bowel Syndrome". *Annals of Clinical Microbiology and Antimicrobials* 13 (1). https://doi.org/10.1186/s12941-014-0049-x

Gatta, L., et. al. 2017. "Systematic review with meta-analysis: Rifaximin is effective and safe for the Treatment of Small intestine Bacterial Overgrowth". *Alimentary Pharmacology & Therapeutics* 45 (5): 604-616. https://doi.org/10.1111/apt.13928

Low, K., et. al. 2010. "A Combination of Rifaximin and Neomycin Is Most Effective in Treating Irritable Bowel Syndrome Patients with Methane on Lactulose Breath Test". *Journal of Clinical Gastroenterology* 44 (8): 547-550. https://doi.org/10.1097/MCG.0b013e3181c64c90

Mayo Clinic staff. 2020. "C. difficile infection". Mayo Foundation. https://www.mayoclinic.org/diseases-conditions/c-difficile/symptoms-causes/syc-20351691

Pimentel, M., et. al. 2017. "Repeat Rifaximin for Irritable Bowel Syndrome: No Clinically Significant Changes in Stool Microbial Antibiotic Sensitivity". *Digestive Diseases and Sciences* 62 (9): 2455–2463. https://doi.org/10.1007/s10620-017-4598-7

Ruscio, M. 2020. "Overuse of Herbal Antimicrobials & Probiotics," [Audio],. https://drruscio.com/overuse-of-herbal-antimicrobials-probiotics/?rfsn=3764788.6a42e9

Shayto, R. H., et. al. 2016. "Use of rifaximin in gastrointestinal and liver diseases". *World Journal of Gastroenterology* 22 (29). https://doi.org/10.3748/wjg.v22.i29.6638

## PROBIOTICS, PREBIOTICS, AND POSTBIOTICS

Achufusi, T. G. O., et. al. 2020. "Small Intestinal Bacterial Overgrowth: Comprehensive Review of Diagnosis, Prevention, and Treatment Methods". *Cureus* 12 (6): e8860. https://doi.org/10.7759/cureus.8860

Bulsiewicz, W. 2020. *Fiber Fueled. The Plant-Based Gut Health Program for Losing Weight, Restoring Your Health, and Optimizing Your Microbiome.* Avery, an imprint of Pinguin Random House LLC, New York. [Kindle] ISBN 9780593084571

Cerdó, T., et. al. 2017. "Probiotic, Prebiotic, and Brain Development". *Nutrients* 9 (11). https://doi.org/10.3390/nu9111247

Ciorba, M. A. 2012. "A Gastroenterologist's Guide to Probiotics". *Clinical Gastroenterology and Hepatology* 10 (9): 960-968. https://doi.org/10.1016/j.cgh.2012.03.024

Fundrazr. n.d. "American Gut". https://fundrazr.com/americangut?ref=ab_7FRxucBoT6o7FRxucBoT6o

Gibson, G. R., et al. 2017. "Expert consensus document: The International Scientific Association for Probiotics and Prebiotics (ISAPP) consensus statement on the definition and scope of prebiotics". *Nature Reviews Gastroenterology & Hepatology* 14 (8):

491-502. https://doi.org/10.1038/nrgastro.2017.75

Mosley, M. 2017. *Clever Guts Diet: How to revolutionize your body from the inside out*. Short Books, London. ISBN 978-1-78072-304-4

National Center for Complementary and Integrative Health. 2019. "Probiotics: What you need to know". National Institutes of Health. https://www.nccih.nih.gov/health/probiotics-what-you-need-to-know

Permutter, D. n.d. "Probiotics: Five core species". https://www.drperlmutter.com/learn/resources/probiotics-five-core-species

The Microsetta Initiative. n.d. "Welcome to the world's largest citizen science microbiome project". American Gut Project and British Gut Project. https://microsetta.ucsd.edu

## BIOFILM

Bjarnsholt, T. 2013. "The role of bacterial biofilms in chronic infections". *Apmis* 121: 1-58. https://doi.org/10.1111/apm.12099

Costerton, B. 2013. "Dr. Bill Costerton: Diagnosing and Treating Biofilm Infections". *Youtube: biofilm*. [Embedded Video]. https://www.youtube.com/watch?v=aXFl_GGW7x8

Deng, Z., et. al. 2020. "Quorum Sensing, Biofilm, and Intestinal Mucosal Barrier: Involvement the Role of Probiotic". *Frontiers in Cellular and Infection Microbiology* 10. https://doi.org/10.3389/fcimb.2020.538077

Kresser, C. 2018. "Biofilm: What it is and how to treat it". https://kresserinstitute.com/biofilm-what-it-is-and-how-to-treat-it

Macfarlane, S., et. al. 2007. "Microbial biofilms in the human gastrointestinal tract". *Journal of Applied Microbiology* 102 (5): 1187-1196. https://doi.org/10.1111/j.1365-2672.2007.03287.x

Von Rosenvinge, E. C., et. al. 2013. "Microbial biofilms and gastrointestinal diseases" *Pathogens and Disease* 67 (1): 25-38. https://doi.org/10.1111/2049-632x.12020

## THE DIGESTIVE SYSTEM

Dworken, J. H. n.d. "Human digestive system". Structures and functions of the human digestive system. Encyclopedia Britannica. https://www.britannica.com/science/human-digestive-system

Sirus, M. 2014. "Function of the Vagus Nerve". https://drsircus.com/general/function-vagus-nerve

## MOUTH, EYES, AND NOSE

Douillard, J. 2016. "Bitter Is Better". https://lifespa.com/bitter-is-better

Dworken, J. H. n.d. "Salivary glands". Structures and functions of the human digestive system. Encyclopedia Britannica. https://www.britannica.com/science/human-digestive-system

Keremi, B., et. al. 2017. "Stress and Salivary Glands". *Current Pharmaceutical Design* 23 (27). https://doi.org/10.2174/1381612823666170215110648

Lee, R. J., et. al. 2014. "Taste receptors in innate immunity". *Cellular and Molecular Life Sciences* 72 (2): 217-236. https://doi.org/10.1007/s00018-014-1736-7

Lu, P. C.-H., et. al. 2017. "Extraoral bitter taste receptors in health and disease". *Journal of General Physiology* 149 (2): 181-197. https://doi.org/10.1085/jgp.201611637

Malamud, D. 2011. "Saliva as a Diagnostic Fluid". *Dental Clinics of North America* 55 (1): 159-178. https://doi.org/10.1016/j.cden.2010.08.004

Natural Eye Care. n.d. "Herbs for indigestion". https://www.naturaleyecare.com/health-conditions/indigestion/indigestion-herbs.asp

Petersen, P. E. 2003. *The World Oral Health Report 2003: Continuous Improvement of Oral Health in the 21st Century: The Approach of the WHO Global Oral Health Programme*. World Health Organization, Switzerland. https://www.who.int/oral_health/media/en/orh_report03_en.pdf?ua=1

World Health Organisation, 2003. "The World Oral Health Report". [PDF]. https://www.who.int/oral_health/media/en/orh_report03_en.pdf

## ESOPHAGUS AND STOMACH

Ash, M. 2011. "The Role of HCL In Gastric Function and Health". https://www.clinical education.org/resources/reviews/the-role-of-hcl-in-gastric-function-and-health

Charles, D. P. n.d. "Polymerase Chain Reaction (PCR) test". eMedicine Health. https://www.emedicine-health.com/pcr_polymerase_chain_reaction_test/article_em.htm

Eske, J. 2020. "How can you naturally increase stomach acid?" https://www.medicalnewstoday.com/articles/how-to-increase-stomach-acid

Kines, K., et. al. 2016. "Nutritional Interventions for Gastroesophageal Reflux, Irritable Bowel Syndrome, and Hypochlorhydria: A Case Report". Integrative Medicine: A Clinician's Journal 15 (4): 49-53. https://www.ncbi.nlm.nih.gov/pmc/articles/PMC4991651

Pimentel, M. 2018. "Q&A with Dr. Mark Pimentel". Interview by Shivan Sarna. *SIBO SOS Speaker Series*. [Transcript] Chronic Condition Rescue. https://join.sibosos.com/page/94100

Ruscio, M. 2020. "Betaine HCl: How To Take This Digestive Aid for Low Stomach Acid". https://drruscio.com/betaine-hcl

Wright, S. 2012. "3 Tests for Low Stomach Acid". https://healthygut.com/3-tests-for-low-stomach-acid

## LIVER

Brody, J. E. 2009. "The Damage of Reflux (Bile, Not Acid)". The New York Times Online. https://www.nytimes.com/2009/06/30/health/30brod.html

Cancer Council Australia. n.d. "Types of Cancer". https://www.cancer.org.au/cancer-information/types-of-cancer/liver-cancer

Cabot, S. 1999. The *Healthy Liver & Bowel Book: Detoxification Strategies for your Liver & Bowel*. SCB International Inc., Arizona. ISBN 0-9673983-0-4

Hepatitis B Foundation. 2012. "Considering the Transmission of HBV Through Tattooing or Piercing". https://www.hepb.org/blog considering-the-trans-mission-of-hbv-through-tattooing-or-piercing

Higuera, V. 2018. "Liver Cyst". https://www.health-line.com/health/liver-cyst

Jafari, S., et. al. 2010. "Tattooing and the risk of transmission of hepatitis C: A systematic review and meta-analysis". *International Journal of Infectious Diseases* 14 (11): e928-e940. https://doi.org/10.1016/j.ijid.2010.03.019

Lee, Y.-S., et. al. 2017. "Understanding Mind-Body Interaction from the Perspective of East Asian Medicine". *Evidence-Based Complementary and Alternative Medicine* 2017: 1-6. https://doi.org/10.1155/2017/7618419

Miliadis, L., et. al. 2010. "Spontaneous rupture of a large non-parasitic liver cyst: a case report". *Journal of Medical Case Reports* 4 (1). https://doi.org/10.1186/1752-1947-4-2

Liver Foundation. n.d. "Liver Disease". Liver Foundation Australia. https://www.liver.org.au/disease

Liver Foundation. n.d. "Not all liver disease is preventable". Liver Foundation Australia. https://www.liver.org.au/health-and-prevention

Mayo Clinic staff. n.d. "Hepatitis B". Mayo Foundation. https://www.mayoclinic.org/diseases-conditions/hepatitis-b/symptoms-causes/syc-20366802

Mayo Clinic staff. n.d., "Liver transplant". Mayo Foundation. https://www.mayoclinic.org/tests-procedures/liver-transplant/about/pac-20384842

Robillard, N. 2013. Fast tract digestion IBS. First edition. Self Health Publishing, USA. [Kindle] ISBN 978-0-9766425-2-7

Traditional Chinse Medicine World Foundation. n.d. "Emotion Commotion. How Emotions Affect Our Well-Being". https://www.tcmworld.org/emotion-commotion

University of Birmingham. 2017. "What can you do to look after your liver?" Future Learn. https://www.futurelearn.com/info/blog/liver-disease

World Cancer Research Fund, and American Institute for Cancer Research. Continuous Update. *Diet, nutrition, physical activity and liver cancer. Project Expert Report 2018*. World Cancer Research Fund International. https://www.wcrf.org/dietandcancer/liver-cancer

World Health Organisation. 2018. "Hepatitis". https://www.who.int/news-room/q-a-detail/hepatitis

### GALLBLADDER

Ballantyne, S. 2012. "The Link Between Gallbladder Disease and Gluten Sensitivity". https://www.thepaleomom.com/the-link-between-gallblad-der-disease-and-gluten-sensitivity

Jacob, Aglaée. 2013. *Digestive Health with REAL Food. A Practical Guide to an Anti-Inflammatory, Low-Irritant, Nutrient-Dense Diet for IBS and Other Digestive Issues*. Paleo Media Group. [Kindle] ISBN 13: 978-0-9887172-0-6

National Institute of Diabetes and Digestive and Kidney Diseases. n.d. "Dieting & Gallstones". National Institute of Health. https://www.niddk.nih.gov/health-information/digestive-diseases/gallstones/dieting

National Institute of Diabetes and Digestive and Kidney Diseases. n.d. "Gallstones". National Institute of Health. https://www.niddk.nih.gov/health-information/digestive-diseases/gallstones

### PANCREAS

Freeman, H. J. 2006. "Hepatobiliary and pancreatic disorders in celiac disease". *World Journal of Gastroenterology* 12 (10): 1503-1508. https://doi.org/10.3748/wjg.v12.i10.1503

John Hopkins Medicine. n.d. "The Digestive Process: What Is the Role of Your Pancreas in Digestion?". https://www.hopkinsmedicine.org/health/conditions-and-diseases/the-digestive-process-what-is-the-role-of-your-pancreas-in-digestion

Diabetes Australia. n.d. "Type 2 diabetes". https://www.diabetesaustralia.com.au/about-diabetes/type-2-diabetes

DiMagno, M. J., et. al. 2013. "Chronic pancreatitis". *Current Opinion in Gastroenterology* 29 (5): 531-536. https://doi.org/10.1097/MOG.0b013e3283639370

Victoria State Government Health. 2014. "Pancreatitis". Better Health Channel. The Department of Health. https://www.betterhealth.vic.gov.au/health/conditionsandtreatments/pancreatitis

### GASTROINTESTINAL CANAL

Brisson, J. 2016. "Can Ingesting Collagen Improve Your Digestive Health?" Fix Your Gut. https://www.fixyourgut.com/can-ingesting-collagen-im-prove-your-digestive-health

Peckham, M. 2004. "Four layers of the G.I. tract". Faculty of Biological Sciences, University of Leeds. https://www.histology.leeds.ac.uk/digestive/GI_lay-ers.php

Santa Cruz, J. 2019. "Dietary Collagen — Should Consumers Believe the Hype?". https://www.todays-dietitian.com/newarchives/0319p26.shtml

Uchida, K., et. al. 2007. "Muscularis mucosae - the forgotten sibling". *Journal of Smooth Muscle Research* 43 (5): 157-177. https://doi.org/10.1540/jsmr.43.157

### SMALL INTESTINE

Dukowicz, A. C., et. al. 2007. "Small intestinal bacterial overgrowth: a comprehensive review". *Gastroenterol Hepatol (NY)* 3 (2): 112-22. https://www.ncbi.nlm.nih.gov/pubmed/21960820

Jacob, Aglaée. 2013. *Digestive Health with REAL Food. A Practical Guide to an Anti-Inflammatory, Low-Irritant, Nutrient-Dense Diet for IBS and Other Digestive Issues*. Paleo Media Group. [Kindle] ISBN 13: 978-0-9887172-0-6

## MIGRATING MOTOR COMPLEX

Deloose, E., et. al. 2012. "The migrating motor complex: control mechanisms and its role in health and disease". Nature Reviews Gastroenterology & Hepatology 9 (5): 271-85. https://doi.org/10.1038/nrgastro.2012.57

Miyano, Y., et. al. 2013. "The Role of the Vagus Nerve in the Migrating Motor Complex and Ghrelin- and Motilin-Induced Gastric Contraction in Suncus". Plos one 8 (5): e64777. https://doi.org/10.1371/journal.pone.0064777

Pimentel, M. 2018. "Q&A with Dr. Mark Pimentel". Interview by Shivan Sarna. SIBO SOS Speaker Series. [Transcript] Chronic Condition Rescue. https://join.sibosos.com/page/94100

## ILEOCECAL VALVE

Hayden, C. n. d. "Digestive System: Ileocecal Valve (ICV) Dysfunction". http://haydeninstitute.com/specific-conditions/digestive-system-ileocecal-valve-icv-dysfunction

Miller, L., et. al. 2012. "Ileocecal valve dysfunction in Small Intestinal Bacterial Overgrowth: A pilot study". World Journal of Gastroenterology 18 (46): 6801–6808. https://doi.org/10.3748/wjg.v18.i46.6801

Rodriguez, D. A., et. al. 2019. "Small Intestinal Bacterial Overgrowth in Children: A State-Of-The-Art Review". Frontiers in Paediatrics. https://doi.org/10.3389/fped.2019.00363

The SIBO Doctor. 2020. "How to release a stuck ileocecal valve". YouTube. [Embedded Video]. https://www.youtube.com/watch?v=ATmSVdeSo_U

The SIBO Doctor. 2020. " How to Release a Stuck Ileocecal Valve - Discussion with Dr Jacobi". YouTube. [Embedded Video]. https://www.youtube.com/watch?v=wdr02kfS7-A

## LARGE INTESTINE

Better Health. n. d. "Pelvic floor". Victoria State Government Australia. https://www.betterhealth.vic.gov.au/health/conditionsandtreatments/pelvic-floor

Cleveland Clinic. n. d. "Pelvic Floor Dysfunction". https://my.clevelandclinic.org/health/diseases/14459-pelvic-floor-dysfunction

International Foundation for Gastrointestinal Disorders. n.d. "Disorders of the large intestine". https://aboutgimotility.org/learn-about-gi-motility/disorders-of-the-large-intestine

Jandhyala, S. M. 2015. "Role of the normal gut microbiota". World Journal of Gastroenterology 21 (29). https://doi.org/10.3748/wjg.v21.i29.8787

Mosley, M. 2017. Clever Guts Diet: How to revolutionize your body from the inside out. Short Books, London. ISBN: 978-1-78072-304-4

The Barral Institute. n.d. "Discover Visceral Manipulation". https://discovervm.com

## MICOBIOME

Palmer, C., et. al. 2007. "Development of the Human Infant Intestinal Microbiota". PLOS Biology. https://doi.org/10.1371/journal.pbio.0050177

## STRESS

Abundant Life Natural Health. n.d. "Safe and Sound Protocol – A comprehensive guide". https://www.anabundantlife.com.au/safe-sound-protocol

Arnsten, A. F. 2009. "Stress signalling pathways that impair prefrontal cortex structure and function". Nat Rev Neurosci 10 (6): 410-22. https://doi.org/10.1038/nrn2648

Canadian Society of Intestinal Research (GI Society). n.d. "Irritable Bowel Syndrome (IBS) and serotonin". https://badgut.org/information-centre/a-z-digestive-topics/ibs-and-serotonin

Cramer, H. et. al. 2017. "Randomised clinical trial: yoga vs written self-care advice for ulcerative colitis". AP&T Alimentary Pharmacology and Therapeutics. https://doi.org/10.1111/apt.14062

Co, S., et. al. 2002. Your hands can heal you. Atria, New York. ISBN 978-0-7432-4305-6

Curlewis, F. n.d. "The founder – Master Choa Kok Sui". Pranic Healing Centre, Brisbane Australia. https://pranichealingcentre.com.au/master-choa-kok-sui

Dienstmann, G. n.d. "Walking meditation — the ultimate guide". Live and Dare. https://liveanddare.com/walking-meditation

European League Against Rheumatism. 2019. "Vagus nerve stimulation study shows significant reduction in rheumatoid arthritis symptoms". https://www.sciencedaily.com/releases/2019/06/190614082931.htm

Gerritsen, R. J. S., et. al. 2018. "Breath of life: The respiratory vagal stimulation model of contemplative activity". Front Hum Neurosci 12: 397. https://doi.org/10.3389/fnhum.2018.00397

Habib, Navaz. 2019. Activate Your Vagus Nerve. Unleash Your Body's Natural Ability to Heal. Ulysses Press, US. [Kindle] ISBN 978-1-61243-910-5

Integrated Listening Australia. n.d. "Safe and Sound protocol". https://aus.integratedlistening.com/safe-and-sound-protocol

Jenkins, T. A., et. al. "Influence of tryptophan and serotonin on mood and cognition with a possible role of the gut-brain axis". Nutrients 8 (1). https://doi.org/10.3390/nu8010056

John Hopkins Medicine. n.d. "Irritable Bowel Syndrome (IBS): Introduction". [PDF]. John Hopkins Medicine Health Library. https://www.hopkinsmedicine.org/gastroenterologyhepatology/_pdfs/small_large_intestine/irritable_bowel_byndrome_IBS.pdf

Koopman, F. A., et. al. 2014. "Vagus nerve stimulation: A new bioelectronics approach to treat rheumatoid arthritis?" Best Practice & Research Clinical Rheumatology 28 (4): 625-635. https://doi.org/10.1016/j.berh.2014.10.015

Kresser, C. 2010. "Chinese medicine demystified (part iv): How acupuncture works". https://chriskresser.com/chinese-medicine-demystified-part-iv-how-acupuncture-works

Kresser, C. 2019. "How Stress Wreaks Havoc on Your Gut – and What to Do about It". https://chriskresser.com/how-stress-wreaks-havoc-on-your-gut

Laborde, S., et. al. 2017. "Heart rate variability and cardiac vagal tone in psychophysiological research - recommendations for experiment planning, data analysis, and data reporting". *Front Psychol* 8: 213. https://doi.org/10.3389/fpsyg.2017.00213

Larauch, M., et. al. 2011. "Stress-Related Alterations of Visceral Sensation: Animal Models for Irritable Bowel Syndrome Study". *J Neurogastroenterol Motil.* https://doi.org/10.5056/jnm.2011.17.3.213

Master Choa Kok Sui. 2004. *Miracles through Pranic Healing. Practical Manual on Energy Healing.* Fourth edition. Institute for Inner Studies Publishing Foundation, Philippines. ISBN 971-0376-04-7

McClain, K. n.d. "Safe and Sound protocol - SSP". Accessed 2019, Dec 8. https://katiemcclain.com/safe-and-sound-protocol-ssp

Plum Village. n.d. "Plum Village". https://plumvillage.org/about/plum-village

Porges, S. W. 2017. *The Pocket Guide to The Polyvagal Theory. The Transformative Power of Feeling Safe.* W.W. Norton & Company, New York. [Kindle] ISBN 978-0-393-70853-0

Porges, S. W. 2009. "The polyvagal theory: new insights into adaptive reactions of the autonomic nervous system". *Cleve Clin J Med* 76 Suppl 2: S86-90. https://doi.org/10.3949/ccjm.76.s2.17

Porges, S. W., et. al. 2011. "The early development of the autonomic nervous system provides a neural platform for social behavior: A polyvagal perspective". *Infant Child Dev* 20 (1): 106-118. https://doi.org/10.1002/icd.688

Porges, S. W. n.d. "An interview with Stephen Porges, PhD. Creator of the Polyvagal Theory". Interview by Ryan Howes. PESI [Blog]. https://www.pesi.com/blog/details/967/wearing-your-heart-on-your-face-the-polyvagal-circuit

Rosenberg, S. 2017. *Accessing The Healing Power of The Vagus Nerve. Self-Help Exercises for Anxiety, Depression, Trauma, And Autism.* North Atlantic Books, California. [Kindle] ISBN 978-1-62317-025-7

Sinha, S. S., et. al. 2018. "Effect of 6 months of meditation on blood sugar, glycosylated hemoglobin, and insulin levels in patients of coronary artery disease". *International Journal of Yoga* 11 (2). https://doi.org/10.4103/ijoy.IJOY_30_17

Stetter, F., et. al. 2002. "Autogenic training: a meta-analysis of clinical outcome studies". *Appl Psychophysiol Biofeedback* 27 (1): 45-98. https://doi.org/10.1023/a:1014576505223

Stasi, C., et. al. 2014. "Serotonin receptors and their role in the pathophysiology and therapy of Irritable Bowel Syndrome". *Techniques in Coloproctology* 18 (7): 613-621. https://doi.org/10.1007/s10151-013-1106-8

Sun, Y., et. al. 2019. "Stress Triggers Flare of Inflammatory Bowel Disease in Children and Adults". *Frontiers in Pediatrics.* https://doi.org/10.3389/fped.2019.00432

Vahora, I. S., et. al. 2020. "How serotonin level fluctuation affects the effectiveness of treatment in Irritable Bowel Syndrome". *Cureus.* https://doi.org/10.7759/cureus.9871

Waxenbaum, J., et. al. 2020. "Anatomy, Autonomic Nervous System". National Center for Biotechnology Information. (NCBI) Bookshelf: Treasure Island (FL). https://www.ncbi.nlm.nih.gov/books/NBK539845

Yi, L. et al. 2017. "Maternal Separation Induced Visceral Hypersensitivity from Childhood to Adulthood". *J Neurogastroenterol Motil.* https://doi.org/10.5056/jnm16089

## MENTAL STRESS

Arnsten, A. F. 2009. "Stress signalling pathways that impair prefrontal cortex structure and function". *Nat Rev Neurosci* 10 (6): 410-22. https://doi.org/10.1038/nrn2648.

Australian Kinesiology Association. n.d. "What is kinesiology? A new healing science comes of age". https://www.aka.asn.au/about-kinesiology

EABP Body Psychotherapy. 2015. "What is Body Psychotherapy?" *YouTube.* [Embedded Video]. https://www.youtube.com/watch?v=04jL4CY-QuM

Feinstein, D. 2012. "Acupoint stimulation in treating psychological disorders: Evidence of efficacy". *Review of General Psychology* 16 (4): 364-380. https://doi.org/10.1037/a0028602

Ford, S. n.d. "Gut-centred hypnotherapy," Interview by Nirala Jacobi. The SIBO Doctor podcast 48. https://www.thesibodoctor.com/2019/09/27/gut-centred-hypnotherapy-sarita-ford-biome-clinic

Institute of Core Energetics. n.d. "A brief autobiography of John C. Pierrakos, M.D". https://www.coreenergetics.org/autobiography-john-pierrakos

iRest. n.d. "iRest Yoga Nidra research". Integrative Restoration Institute. https://www.irest.org/irest-research

Miller, J. A. 2010. "Alexander Lowen (1910–2008): reflections on his life". *Body, Movement and Dance in Psychotherapy* 5 (2): 197-202. https://doi.org/10.1080/17432979.2010.494854

Miller, R. 2015. "Reflections on teaching meditation, Richard Miller". Science and Nonduality. *YouTube.* [Embedded Video]. https://www.youtube.com/watch?v=dx4jar_PMkl

Miller, R. 2015, May 21. "Reflections on the path to healing, Richard Miller". Science and Nonduality. *YouTube.* [Embedded Video]. https://www.youtube.com/watch?v=ZPM0vJmOTXA

Mind + Gut clinic Australia. n.d. "Treatments". https://www.mindgutclinic.com.au/treatments.html

Nk Institute. n.d. "History of Kinesiology". https://www.nkinstitute.com.au/history-of-kinesiology.html

Peters, S. 2017. "How effective is Gut-Directed Hypnotherapy in People with IBS?" Monash University Australia, FODMAP blog. https://www.monashfodmap.com/blog/how-effective-is-gut-directed

Peters, S., et. al. n.d. "How hypnotherapy is helping treat Irritable Bowel Syndrome

(IBS) sufferers". https://lens.monash.edu/@medicine-health/2019/06/24/1351605/how-hypnotherapy-is-helping-people-suffering-from-irritable-bowel-syndrome-ibs

The Alexander Lowen Foundation. n.d. "Alexander Lowen M.D. (1910 - 2008)". https://www.lowenfoundation.org/about-alexander-lowen

Van Susteren, L., et. al. 2020. *Emotional Inflammation. Discover Your Triggers and Reclaim Your Equilibrium During Anxious Times.* Sounds True. [Kindle] ISBN: 9781683644569

### DIETARY STRESS

David, M. 2005. *The Slow Down Diet: Eating for Pleasure, Energy, and Weight Loss.* Healing Arts Press, Vermont US. [Kindle] ISBN 978-1-62055-509-5

OCD Center of Los Angeles, Carlifonia. 2019. "Orthorexia: Where eating disorders meet OCD". http://ocdla.com/orthorexia-eating-disorders-ocd-1977

### EXERCISE

Johannesson, E., et. al. 2011. "Physical Activity Improves Symptoms in Irritable Bowel Syndrome: A Randomized Controlled Trial". *American Journal of Gastroenterology* 106 (5): 915-922. https://doi.org/10.1038/ajg.2010.480

De Oliveira, E. P., et. al. 2014. "Gastrointestinal Complaints During Exercise: Prevalence, Etiology, and Nutritional Recommendations". *Sports Medicine* 44 (S1): 79-85. https://doi.org/10.1007/s40279-014-0153-2

Canadian Society of Intestinal Research (GI Society). n.d. "Physical activity and digestive health: It's complicated!" https://badgut.org/information-centre/a-z-digestive-topics/physical-activity-and-gi-health

### SLEEP

Bertrand, P., et. al. 2016. "Gut feeling: how your Microbiota affects your Mood, Sleep and Stress Levels". https://theconversation.com/gut-feeling-how-your-microbiota-affects-your-mood-sleep-and-stress-levels-65107

Boudjeltia, K. Z., et. al. 2008. "Sleep restriction increases white blood cells, mainly neutrophil count, in young healthy men: A pilot study". *Vascular Health Risk Management* 4 (6). 1467-1470. https://doi.org/10.2147/vhrm.s3934

Erickson Gabbey, A. 2019. "What Are Biological Rhythms?". https://www.healthline.com/health/biological-rhythms

Harvard Health Publishing. 2018. "Blue light has a dark side". Harvard Medical School. https://www.health.harvard.edu/staying-healthy/blue-light-has-a-dark-side

Galland, L. 2014. "The Gut Microbiome and the Brain". *Journal of Medicinal Food* 17 (12): 1261-1272. https://doi.org/10.1089/jmf.2014.7000

NCCIH Clearinghouse, PubMD. n.d. "Melatonin: What you need to know". https://www.nccih.nih.gov/health/melatonin-what-you-need-to-know

Mandal, A. 2019. "What are Cytokines?". https://www.news-medical.net/health/What-are-Cytokines.aspx

Mullington, J. M., et. al. 2010. "Sleep Loss and Inflammation". *Best Practice & Research Clinical Endocrinology Metabolism.* 24(5): 775–784. https://doi.org/10.1016/j.beem.2010.08.014

Rrince, R. 2021. "How sleeps works". One Care Media. https://www.sleep.org/how-sleep-works

Sleep Health Foundation Australia. 2011. "Insomnia". https://www.sleephealthfoundation.org.au/insomnia.html

Scott, T. 2011. *The Anti-Anxiety Food Solution. How the Food You Eat Can Help You Calm Your Anxious Mind, Improve Your Mood and End Cravings.* Viking Penguin a division of Penguin Group (USA) Inc., ISBN: 978-1-57224-925-7 (Pbk)

Scott, T. 2020. "GABA and Tryptophan for Anxiety and Insomnia". Interview by Misty Williams. *Your Best Sleep Ever! Summit.* https://7day.healthmeans.com/slp20

Wallis, A., et. al. 2016. "Support for the Microgenderome: Associations in a Human Clinical Population". *Scientific Reports* 6 (1). https://doi.org/10.1038/srep19171

### INFLAMMATION

Elmer, J. 2018. "Inflammation: What You Need to Know". https://www.healthline.com/health/inflammation#diagnosis

Calder, P.C., et. al. 2009. "Inflammatory Disease Processes and Interactions with Nutrition". *British Journal of Nutrition,* 101 (S1):1 – 45. https://doi.org/10.1017/S0007114509377867

Bonaccio, M., et. al. 2017. "Mediterranean Diet, Dietary Polyphenols and Low-Grade Inflammation: Results from the MOLI-SANI study". *British Journal of Clinical Pharmacology* 83 (1): 107-113. https://doi.org/10.1111/bcp.12924

McManus. K. 2020. "Do pro-inflammatory diets harm our health? And can anti-inflammatory diets help?" Harvards Health Puplishing. https://www.health.harvard.edu/blog/do-pro-inflammatory-diets-harm-our-health-and-can-anti-inflammatory-diets-help-2020122321624

Minihane, A. M., et. al. 2015. "Low-grade inflammation, diet composition and health: current research evidence and its translation". *British Journal of Nutrition* 114 (7): 999-1012. https://doi.org/10.1017/s0007114515002093

Szalay, J. 2018. "What Is Inflammation?". https://www.livescience.com/52344-inflammation.html

Watson. J., et. al. 2019. "Use of multiple inflammatory marker tests in primary care: using Clinical Practice Research Datalink to evaluate accuracy". *British Journal of General Practice* 69 (684): e462-e460. https://doi.org/10.3399/bjgp19X704309

## MICROPLASTIC

Calderwood, I. 2018. "16 times countries and cities have banned single-use plastics". Global Poverty Project. https://www.globalcitizen.org/en/content/plastic-bans-around-the-world

Cox, K. D., et. al. 2019. "Human consumption of microplastics". *Environmental Science & Technology* 53 (12): 7068-7074. https://doi.org/10.1021/acs.est.9b01517

Gibbens, S. 2019. "You eat thousands of bits of Plastic every Year. Though abundant in Water, Air, and common Foods, it's unclear how it might affect our Health". https://www.nationalgeographic.com/environment/article/microplastics-found-90-percent-table-salt-sea-salt

Karami, A., et. al. 2017. "The presence of microplastics in commercial salts from different countries". *Scientific Reports* 7 (1). https://doi.org/10.1038/srep46173

Kim, J.-S., et. al. 2018. "Global pattern of microplastics (MPs) in commercial food-grade salts: Sea salt as an indicator of seawater mp pollution". *Environmental Science & Technology* 52 (21): 12819-12828. https://doi.org/10.1021/acs.est.8b04180

Leman, J. 2018. "Car tires and brake pads produce harmful microplastics. These particles can end up in bodies of freshwater and, eventually, the ocean". Society for Science & the Public. https://www.sciencenews.org/article/car-tires-and-brake-pads-produce-harmful-microplastics

Liebezeit, G., et. al. 2013. "Non-pollen particulates in honey and sugar". *Food Addit Contam Part A Chem Anal Control Expo Risk Assess* 30 (12): 2136-40. https://doi.org/10.1080/19440049.2013.843025

Mayo Clinic staff. n.d. "What is BPA, and what are the concerns about BPA?" Mayo Foundation. https://www.mayoclinic.org/healthy-lifestyle/nutrition-and-healthy-eating/expert-answers/bpa/faq-20058331

Parker, L. 2018. "Microplastics found in 90 percent of table salt. A new study looked at sea, rock, and lake salt sold around the world. Here's what you need to know". https://www.nationalgeographic.com/environment/article/microplastics-found-90-percent-table-salt-sea-salt

Pfeifer, H. 2018. "The UK now has one of world's toughest microbead bans". Cable News Network, Health. http://edition.cnn.com/2018/01/09/health/microbead-ban-uk-intl/index.html

Plastic Soup Foundation. 2019. "Start of Scientific Research into the Health Risks of Microplastics: Does Plastic make us sick?" https://www.plasticsoupfoundation.org/en/2019/02/scientific-research-into-health-risks-of-microplastics-does-plastic-make-us-sick

Rößiger, M. 2018. "Pestizide, Weichmacher, Aromaten: Die giftige Fracht im Mikroplastik". Spectum. https://www.spektrum.de/news/die-giftige-fracht-im-mikroplastik/1585272

Schulz, M. 2018. "NDR - research shows: Especially the high-priced salt Fleur de Sel contains plastic". RHEWUM GmbH. https://www.rhewum.com/news/715/254/NDR-research-shows-Especially-the-high-priced-salt-Fleur-de-Sel-contains-plastic.html

Smith, M., et. al. 2018. "Microplastics in Seafood and the Implications for Human Health". *Curr Environ Health Rep* 5 (3): 375-386. https://doi.org/10.1007/s40572-018-0206-z

Sommer, F., et. al. 2018. "Tire abrasion as a major source of microplastics in the environment". *Aerosol and Air Quality Research* 18 (8): 2014-2028. https://doi.org/10.4209/aaqr.2018.03.0099

Spink Health. 2018. "Microplastics discovered in human stools across the globe in 'first study of its kind'". The American Association for Advancement of Science. EurekAlert! https://www.eurekalert.org/pub_releases/2018-10/sh-mdi101518.php

Technical University Munich. 2019. "How dangerous is microplastic?". https://phys.org/news/2019-01-dangerous-microplastic.html

Thompson, R. C., et. al. 2009. "Plastics, the environment and human health: current consensus and future trends". *Philos Trans R Soc Lond B Biol Sci* 364 (1526): 2153-66. https://doi.org/10.1098/rstb.2009.0053

Toussaint, B., et. al. 2019. "Review of micro- and nanoplastic contamination in the food chain". *Food Additives & Contaminants: Part A* 36 (5): 639-673. https://doi.org/10.1080/19440049.2019.1583381

Wright, S. L., et. al. 2017. "Plastic and human health: A micro issue?" *Environmental Science & Technology* 51 (12): 6634-6647. https://doi.org/10.1021/acs.est.7b00423

Yang, D., et. al. 2015. "Microplastic pollution in table salts from china". *Environ Sci Technol* 49 (22): 13622-7. https://doi.org/10.1021/acs.est.5b03163

## IMMUNE SYSTEM

Ballantyne, S. 2014. "Which comes first: the leaky gut or the dysfunctional immune system?" https://www.thepaleomom.com/comes-first-leaky-gut-dysfunctional-immune-system/?cn-reloaded=1

Belkaid, Y., et. al. 2014. "Role of the Microbiota in Immunity and Inflammation". *Cell* 157 (1): 121-141. https://doi.org/10.1016/j.cell.2014.03.011

Blach-Olszewska, Z., et. al. 2007. "Mechanisms of over-activated innate immune system regulation in autoimmune and neurodegenerative disorders". *Neuropsychiatr Dis Treat.* 3 (3): 365–372. https://www.ncbi.nlm.nih.gov/pmc/articles/PMC2654796

Callier, V. 2016. "Autoimmune diseases may be side effect of a strong immune system". https://www.newscientist.com/article/2099313-autoimmune-diseases-may-be-side-effect-of-a-strong-immune-system

The National Institute of Environmental Health Sciences. n.d. "Autoimmune Diseases". https://www.niehs.nih.gov/health/topics/conditions/autoimmune/index.cfm

## IMMUNOGLOBULIN

American Academy of Allery, Asthma and Immunology. 2020 "Food intolerance versus food allergy". https://www.aaaai.org/Tools-for-the-Public/Conditions-Library/Allergies/food-intolerance

American Academy of Allery, Asthma and Immunology. 2020 "The myth of IgG food panel testing". https://www.aaaai.org/Tools-for-the-Public/Conditions-Library/Allergies/IgG-food-test

Cedars Sinai. n.d. "IgG deficiencies". The Stay Well Company. https://www.cedars-sinai.org/health-library/diseases-and-conditions/i/igg-deficiencies.html

Lim, H.-S., et. al. 2018. "Food elimination diet and nutritional deficiency in patients with inflammatory bowel disease". Clinical Nutrition Research 7 (1). https://doi.org/10.7762/cnr.2018.7.1.48

Lab Tests Online Australasia. n.d. "Immunoglobulins". https://www.labtestsonline.org.au/learning/test-index/quantitative-immunoglobulins

Masu, Y., et. al. 2021. "Immunoglobulin subtype-coated bacteria are correlated with the disease activity of inflammatory bowel disease". Scientific Reports 11 Article number: 16672. https://www.nature.com/articles/s41598-021-96289-5

Mazzocchi, A., et. al. 2017. "The role of nutritional aspects in food allergy: Prevention and management". Nutrients 9 (8). https://doi.org/10.3390/nu9080850

## LEAKY GUT

Baily, C. 2014. "Cyrex testing: What you need to know". https://www.christinebailey.co.uk/cyrex-testing-what-you-need-to-know

Ballantyne, S. 2013. The Paleo Approach: Reverse Autoimmune Disease and Heal Your Body. p. 53-60. Las Vegas: Victory Belt Publishing Inc. ISBN 978-1-936608-39-3

Bulsiewicz, W. 2020. Fiber Fueled. The Plant-Based Gut Health Program for Losing Weight, Restoring Your Health, and Optimizing Your Microbiome. Avery, an imprint of Pinguin Random House LLC, New York. [Kindle] ISBN 9780593084571

Fasano, A. 2012. "Intestinal Permeability and Its Regulation by Zonulin: Diagnostic and Therapeutic Implications". Clinical Gastroenterology and Hepatology 10 (10): 1096-1100. https://doi.org/10.1016/j.cgh.2012.08.012

Groschwitz, K. R., et. al. 2009. "Intestinal barrier function: Molecular regulation and disease pathogenesis". Journal of Allergy and Clinical Immunology 124 (1): 3-20. https://doi.org/10.1016/j.jaci.2009.05.038

Li, H., et al. 2015. "The outer mucus layer hosts a distinct intestinal microbial niche". Nature Communications 6 (1). https://doi.org/10.1038/ncomms9292

Johansson, M. E., et. al. 2013. "The gastrointestinal mucus system in health and disease". Nat Rev Gastroenterol Hepatol 10 (6): 352-61.

https://doi.org/10.1038/nrgastro.2013.35

Kresser, C. 2018. "The Clinical Utility of Zonulin Testing?". https://kresserinstitute.com/clinical-utility-zonulin-testing

Krishnan, K. 2021. "How to achieve total gut restoration with Kiran Krishnan (Updated with Q&A)". [Video] https://sibosos.com/how-to-achieve-total-gut-restoration-with-kiran-krishnan

Mu, Q., et. al. 2017. "Leaky gut as a danger signal for autoimmune diseases". Frontiers in Immunology 8. https://doi.org/10.3389/fimmu.2017.00598

NutriPATH. n.d. "Intestinal permeability – 6 hour urine". https://www.nutripath.com.au/product/intestinal-permeability-urine-test-code-2011

NutriPATH. n.d. "Zonulin- faecal". https://www.nutripath.com.au/product/zonulin-blood-test-code-2023

Wu, H. J., et. al. "The role of gut microbiota in immune homeostasis and autoimmunity". Gut Microbes 3 (1): 4-14. https://doi.org/10.4161/gmic.19320.

Zhou, Q., et. al. 2019. "Randomised placebo-controlled trial of dietary glutamine supplements for postinfectious Irritable Bowel Syndrome". Gut 68 (6): 996-1002. https://doi.org/10.1136/gutjnl-2017-315136

## HISTAMINE

Aha! Swiss Allergy Centre. n.d. "Histamine intolerance". https://www.aha.ch/swiss-allergy-centre/allergies-intolerances/food-intolerances/histamine-intolerance

Branco, A. C. C. C., et. al. 2018. "Role of histamine in modulating the immune response and inflammation". Mediators of Inflammation 2018: 1-10. https://doi.org/10.1155/2018/9524075

Kresser, C. 2019. "Could your histamine intolerance really be mast cell activation disorder?". https://chriskresser.com/could-your-histamine-intolerance-really-be-mast-cell-activation-disorder

Maintz, L., et. al. 2007. "Histamine and histamine intolerance". The American Journal of Clinical Nutrition 85 (5): 1185-1196. https://doi.org/10.1093/ajcn/85.5.1185

Reese, I., et. al. 2017. "German guideline for the management of adverse reactions to ingested histamine". Allergo Journal International 26 (2): 72-79. https://doi.org/10.1007/s40629-017-0011-5

Ruscio, M. 2020. "How to use a low histamine diet for histamine intlerance". https://drruscio.com/low-histamine-diet

The SIBO Doctor. n.d. "Get started with Dr Jacobi's Bi-Phasic approach". [PDF]. https://www.thesibodoctor.com/sibo-bi-phasic-diet-free-downloads

The SIBO Doctor. SIBO/Histamine. [PDF]. https://www.thesibodoctor.com/histamine-sibo-bi-phasic-diet

## OXALATES

Arnarson, A. 2017. "How to reduce antinutrients in foods". https://www.healthline.com/nutrition/how-to-reduce-antinutrients

Holmes, R. P., et. al. 2001. "Contribution of dietary oxalate to urinary oxalate excretion". *Kidney International* 59 (1):270-6. https://doi.org/10.1046/j.1523-1755.2001.00488.x

Holmes, R. P., et. al. 2000. "Estimation of the oxalate content of foods and daily oxalate intake". *Kidney International* 57 (4): 1662-1667. https://doi.org/10.1046/j.1523-1755.2000.00010.x

Liebman, M., et. al. 2011. "Probiotics and other key determinants of dietary oxalate absorption". *Advances in Nutrition* 2 (3): 254-260. https://doi.org/10.3945/an.111.000414

Morrison, S. C., et. al. 2003. "Oxalates". In *Encyclopedia of Food Sciences and Nutrition*, 4282-4287. https://doi.org/10.1016/b0-12-227055-x/01378-x

Noonan, S. C., et. al. 1999. "Oxalate content of foods and its effect on humans". *Asia Pacific Journal of Clinical Nutrition* 8 (1): 64-74. https://doi.org/10.1046/j.1440-6047.1999.00038.x

Rostenberg, A. 2016. "Oxalates and MTHFR: Understanding the gut-kidney axis". Beyond MTHFR. https://www.beyondmthfr.com/oxalates-and-mthfr-understanding-the-gut-kidney-axis

Savage, G. P., et. al. 2009. "The effect of soaking and cooking on the oxalate content of taro leaves". *International Journal of Food Sciences and Nutrition* 57 (5-6): 376-381. https://doi.org/10.1080/09637480600855239

Shaw, W. 2015. "The green smoothie fad: This road to health hell is paved with toxic oxalate crystals". https://www.townsendletter.com/Jan2015/green0115.html

Tang, M., et. al. 2008. "Effect of cinnamon and turmeric on urinary oxalate excretion, plasma lipids, and plasma glucose in healthy subjects". *The American Journal of Clinical Nutrition* 87 (5): 1262-1267. https://doi.org/10.1093/ajcn/87.5.1262

The Great Plains Laboratory. 2016. "Oxalates". https://www.greatplainslaboratory.com/gpl-blog-source/2016/8/8/oxalates

## SALICYLATES

Baenkler, H.-W. 2008. "Salicylate intolerance". *Deutsches Aerzteblatt Online*. https://doi.org/10.3238/arztebl.2008.0137

Beck, D. n.d. "Salicylate sensitivity and SIBO," Interview by Nirala Jacobi. The SIBO Doctor Podcast 4. [Audio]. https://www.thesibodoctor.com/2017/02/02/the-sibo-doctor-podcast-episode-4-salicylate-sensitivity/?v=6cc98ba2045f

Beck, D. 2016. "Salicylate sensitivity: The other food intolerance". ND News & Review. https://ndnr.com/autoimmuneallergy-medicine/salicylate-sensitivity-the-other-food-intolerance

Dengate, S. n.d. "Food intolerance network". https://www.fedup.com.au

WebMD. 2020. "Salicylate allergy". https://www.webmd.com/allergies/salicylate-allergy

WebMD. n.d. "Wintergreen". https://www.webmd.com/vitamins/ai/ingredientmono-783/wintergreen

World Health Organization. 2019. "WHO model list of essential medicines". https://www.who.int/groups/expert-committee-on-selection-and-use-of-essential-medicines/essential-medicines-lists

Yartsev, A. n.d. "Salicylate overdose". https://derangedphysiology.com/main/cicm-primary-exam/required-reading/acid-base-physiology/acid-base-disturbances/Chapter%20619/salicylate-overdose

## CARBOHYDRATES

Barrett, J. 2016. "What are the oligos (Fructans & GOS)?" Monash University Australia, FODMAP blog. https://www.monashfodmap.com/blog/what-are-oligos

Barrett, J, et. al. 2016. "What are polyols?" Monash University Australia, FODMAP blog. https://www.monashfodmap.com/blog/what-are-polyols

Belluz, J. 2018. "A carb called Fructan may be the real culprit behind gluten sensitivity". Vox Media. https://www.vox.com/2017/11/21/16643816/gluten-bloated-carb-wheat-fructan-problem-fodmaps

Cozma-Petrut, A., et. al. 2017. "Diet in Irritable Bowel Syndrome: What to recommend, not what to forbid to patients!" *World J Gastroenterol* 23 (21): 3771-3783. https://doi.org/10.3748/wjg.v23.i21.3771

Esmaillzadeh, A., et. al. 2017. "Consumption of a low fermentable oligo-, di-, mono-saccharides, and polyols diet and Irritable Bowel Syndrome: A systematic review". International Journal of Preventive Medicine 8 (1). https://doi.org/10.4103/ijpvm.IJPVM_175_17

Gibson, P. R., et. al. 2010. "Evidence-based dietary management of functional gastrointestinal symptoms: The FODMAP approach". *Journal of Gastroenterology and Hepatology* 25 (2): 252-258. https://doi.org/10.1111/j.1440-1746.2009.06149.x

Jbpub. 2015. Carbohydrate: Simple sugars and complex chains. Chapter 4. http://samples.jbpub.com/9781284064650/9781284086379_CH04_Disco.pdf

Monash University. 2019. "FODMAPs and Irritable Bowel Syndrome". Monash University Australia, FODMAP blog. https://www.monashfodmap.com/about-fodmap-and-ibs

Specialists in Gastroenterology (SIG). n.d. "Low FODMAP Diet". https://www.gidoctor.net/contents/low-fodmap-diet

Youdim, A., et. al. 2019. "Carbohydrates, Proteins, and Fats". MSD Manual Consumer Version. https://www.msdmanuals.com/en-au/home/disorders-of-nutrition/overview-of-nutrition/carbohydrates,-proteins,-and-fats?redirectid=393

## PROTEIN

Ahmed, T., et. al. 2010. "Assessment and management of nutrition in older people and its importance to health". *Clin Interv Aging* 5: 207-16. https://doi.org/10.2147/cia.s9664

Australian Government. n.d. "Protein". National Health and Medical Research Council. https://www.nrv.gov.au/nutrients/protein

De Angelis, M., et. al. 2020. "Diet influences the functions of the human intestinal microbiome". *Scientific Reports* 10 (1). https://doi.org/10.1038/s41598-020-61192-y

Delimaris, I. 2013. "Adverse effects associated with protein intake above the recommended dietary allowance for adults". *ISRN Nutr* 2013: 126929. https://doi.org/10.5402/2013/126929

Desmond, A. 2020. "Gut And microbiome with Dr. Alan Desmond," Interview by Clint Paddison. *Rheumatoid solution*. [Audio/ Video/ Transcript]. https://www.rheumatoidsolutions.com/gut-and-microbiome-with-dr-alan-desmond

Douillard, J. 2020. "Are you protein deficient? The hidden signs". https://lifespa.com/protein-deficiency-the-hidden-signs

EAT - Lancet Commission. 2019. *Food Planet Health. Healthy diets from sustainable food systems.* [PDF] EAT - Lancet Commission. https://eatforum.org/content/uploads/2019/07/EAT-Lancet_Commission_Summary_Report.pdf

Gebhardt, E., et. al. 2002. "Nutritive value of food". [PDF]. U.S. Department of Agriculture, Agricultural Research. https://www.ars.usda.gov/is/np/NutritiveValueofFoods/NutritiveValueofFoods.pdf

Harvard Health Publishing. 2020. "When it comes to protein, how much is too much?" Harvard Medical School. https://www.health.harvard.edu/nutrition/when-it-comes-to-protein-how-much-is-too-much

Harvard T.H. Chan. n.d. "Protein". School of Public Health. https://www.hsph.harvard.edu/nutritionsource/what-should-you-eat/protein

Lonnie, M., et. al., 2018. "Protein for life: Review of optimal protein intake, sustainable dietary sources and the effect on appetite in ageing adults". *Nutrients* 10 (3). https://doi.org/10.3390/nu10030360

Marsh, K. A., et. al. 2012. "Protein and vegetarian diets". *The Medical Journal of Australia* 1 (2): 7-10. https://www.mja.com.au/system/files/issues/196_10_040612_supplement/mar11492_fm.pdf

MedlinePlus. 2009. "Protein S deficiency". U.S. National Library of Medicine. https://medlineplus.gov/genetics/condition/protein-s-deficiency

MedlinePlus. 2020. Protein C and Protein S tests. U.S. National Library of Medicine. https://medlineplus.gov/lab-tests/protein-c-and-protein-s-tests

Miller, K. 2020. "Muehrcke's lines of the fingernails". https://www.webmd.com/skin-problems-and-treatments/guide/muehrcke-lines-of-the-fingernails

National Research Council (US) Subcommittee. 1989. *Recommended Dietary Allowances. Protein and Amino Acids.* 10th edition ed. NCBI Bookshelf: National Academies Press (US). https://www.ncbi.nlm.nih.gov/books/NBK234922

Oso, A. A., et. al. 2020. "Nutritional Composition of Grain and Seed Proteins". *IntechOpen*. https://doi.org/10.5772/intechopen.97878

Searchinger, T., et. al. 2018, Dec. World resources report. Creating a sustainable food future. A menu of solutions to feed nearly 10 billion people by 2050. World Resources Institute. https://www.wri.org/research/creating-sustainable-food-future

Singal, A., et. al. 2015. "Nail as a window of systemic diseases". *Indian Dermatol Online J* 6 (2): 67-74. https://doi.org/10.4103/2229-5178.153002

Tomova, A., et. al. 2019. "The effects of vegetarian and vegan diets on gut microbiota". *Front Nutr* 6: 47. https://doi.org/10.3389/fnut.2019.00047

Troy, E. 2014. "What is the Difference Between Broth, Stock, and Consommé?". https://culinarylore.com/cooking-terms:difference-between-broth-and-consomme

Youdim, A., et. al. 2019. "Carbohydrates, Proteins, and Fats". MSD Manual Consumer Version. https://www.msdmanuals.com/en-au/home/disorders-of-nutrition/overview-of-nutrition/carbohydrates,-proteins,-and-fats?redirectid=393

## FATS AND OILS

Bancroft, A. 2019. "Cooking with Fats and Oils: Can they withstand the heat?" Colorado State University. Kendall Reagan Nutrition. https://www.chhs.colostate.edu/krnc/monthly-blog/cooking-with-fats-and-oil

Brigham and Women's Hospital. 2021. "Diabetes powerfully associated with premature coronary heart disease in women". https://www.sciencedaily.com/releases/2021/01/210120114835.htm

Bulsiewicz, W. 2020. *Fiber Fueled. The Plant-Based Gut Health Program for Losing Weight, Restoring Health, and Optimizing Your Microbiome.* Avery - an imprint of Penguin Random House, New York. [Kindle] ISBN 978059084571

European Society of Cardiology. 2018. "Too much of a good thing? Very high levels of 'good' cholesterol may be harmful". https://www.sciencedaily.com/releases/2018/08/180825081724.htm

Feingold, K. R. n. d. "Introduction to Lipids and Lipoproteins". https://www.ncbi.nlm.nih.gov/books/NBK305896

Harvard Health Publishing. n.d. "The truth about fats: the good, the bad, and the in-between". Harvard Medical School. https://www.health.harvard.edu/staying-healthy/the-truth-about-fats-bad-and-good

Harvard Health Publishing. 2019. "How it's made: Cholesterol production in your body" Harvard Medical School. https://www.health.harvard.edu/heart-health/how-its-made-cholesterol-production-in-your-body

Harvard Health Publishing. 2020. "Take control of rising cholesterol at menopause". Harvard Medical School. https://www.health.harvard.edu/womens-health/take-control-of-rising-cholesterol-at-menopause

Harvard T.H. Chan. 2021. "Types of fat". Harvard Medical School. https://www.hsph.harvard.edu/nutritionsource/what-should-you-eat/fats-and-cholesterol/types-of-fat

Hightower, N. C., et. al. 2020. "Fats". Encyclopedia Britannica. https://www.britannica.com/science/human-digestive-system/Fats#ref294177

Huff, T., et. al. 2021. *Physiology, cholesterol*. NCBI Bookshelf. StatPearls Publishing. https://www.ncbi.nlm.nih.gov/books/NBK470561

Lenicek, M., et. al. 2011. "Bile acid malabsorption in inflammatory bowel disease: assessment by serum markers". *Inflamm Bowel Dis* 17 (6): 1322-7. https://doi.org/10.1002/ibd.21502

Liu, A. G., et. al. 2017. "A healthy approach to dietary fats: understanding the science and taking action to reduce consumer confusion". *Nutr J* 16 (1): 53. https://doi.org/10.1186/s12937-017-0271-4

Mayo Clinic staff. 2018. "Identifying diarrhea caused by bile acid malabsorption". Mayo Foundation. https://www.mayoclinic.org/medical-professionals/digestive-diseases/news/identifying-diarrhea-caused-by-bile-acid-malabsorption/mac-20430098

McCarthy, K. 2018. "The three classifications of lipids found in food and in the human body". https://healthyeating.sfgate.com/three-classifications-lipids-found-food-human-body-11865.html

National Research Council (US) Committee on Diet and Health. 1989. *Fats and other lipids*. National Academies Press (US). https://www.ncbi.nlm.nih.gov/books/NBK218759

Rahmany, S., and I. Jialal. 2020. *Biochemistry, chylomicron*. NCBI Bookshelf. StatPearls Publishing. https://www.ncbi.nlm.nih.gov/books/NBK545157

Sacks, F. M., et. al. 2017. "Dietary fats and cardiovascular disease: A Presidential Advisory From the American Heart Association". *Circulation* 136 (3): e1-e23. https://doi.org/10.1161/CIR.0000000000000510

SEER training team. 2020. "Introduction to the lymphatic system". NIH, National Cancer Institute. SEER Training Modules. https://training.seer.cancer.gov/anatomy/lymphatic

Slattery, S. A., et. al. 2015. "Systematic review with meta-analysis: the prevalence of bile acid malabsorption in the Irritable Bowel Syndrome with diarrhoea". *Aliment Pharmacol Ther* 42 (1): 3-11. https://doi.org/10.1111/apt.13227

Zaidel, O., et. al. 2003. "Uninvited guests: The impact of Small Intestinal Bacterial Overgrowth on nutritional status". Nutrition Issues in Gastroenterology, Series #7. https://med.virginia.edu/ginutrition/wp-content/uploads/sites/199/2015/11/zaidelarticle-July-03.pdf

Zuvarox, T., et. al. 2021, March 8. *Malabsorption syndromes*. NCBI Bookshelf. StatPearls Publishing. https://www.ncbi.nlm.nih.gov/books/NBK553106

**SATURATED FAT**

Khan Academy Biology. 2015. "Saturated fats, unsaturated fats, and trans fats" *Youtube*. [Embedded Video]. https://www.youtube.com/watch?v=O9lL2KStW9s

Mayo Clinic staff. n. d. "Dietary fat: Know which to choose". Nutrition and healthy eating. https://www.mayoclinic.org/healthy-lifestyle/nutrition-and-healthy-eating/in-depth/fat/art-20045550

Sacks, F. M., et. al. 2017. "Dietary Fats and Fardiovascular Disease: A Presidential Advisory From the American Heart Association". *Circulation* 136 (3): e1-e23. https://doi.org/10.1161/CIR.0000000000000510

**COCONUT OIL**

A&A Pharmachern. 2019. " MCT Oil & MCT Oil Powder. What's the difference?" https://aapharmachem.com/mct-oil-and-oil-powder

Eyres, L., et. al. 2016. "Coconut oil consumption and cardiovascular risk factors in humans". *Nutr Rev* 74 (4): 267-80. https://doi.org/10.1093/nutrit/nuw002

Harvard T.H. Chan. 2021. "Coconut oil". Harvard Medical School. https://www.hsph.harvard.edu/nutritionsource/food-features/coconut-oil

Harvard T.H. Chan. 2021. "Types of fat". Harvard Medical School. https://www.hsph.harvard.edu/nutritionsource/what-should-you-eat/fats-and-cholesterol/types-of-fat

Krishnan, K. 2019. "Supporting the vaginal microbiome, the root cause of acne, & why your dog has leaky gut" Interview by Dhru Purohit. *YouTube*. [Embedded Video]. https://www.youtube.com/watch?v=zUri4cqUVP4

O'Brien, S. 2020. "Science-based benefits of MCT oil". https://www.healthline.com/nutrition/mct-oil-benefits

U.S. Department of agriculture. 2019. "Oil, coconut". U.S. Department of Agriculture (USDA). https://fdc.nal.usda.gov/fdc-app.html#/food-details/330458/nutrients

**UNSATURATED FAT**

Abdullah, M. M. H., et. al. 2017. "Health benefits and evaluation of healthcare cost savings if oils rich in monounsaturated fatty acids were substituted for conventional dietary oils in the United States". *Nutrition Reviews* 75 (3): 163–174. https://doi.org/10.1093/nutrit/nuw062

Bancroft, A. 2019. "Cooking with Fats and Oils: Can they withstand the heat?" Colorado State University. Kendall Reagan Nutrition. https://www.chhs.colostate.edu/krnc/monthly-blog/cooking-with-fats-and-oils

Benbrook, C. M., et. al., 2018. "Enhancing the fatty acid profile of milk through forage-based rations, with nutrition modeling of diet outcomes". *Food Science & Nutrition* 6 (3): 681-700. https://doi.org/10.1002/fsn3.610

Costantini, L., et. al. 2017. "Impact of omega-3 fatty acids on the gut microbiota". *Int J Mol Sci* 18 (12). https://doi.org/10.3390/ijms18122645

Douillard, J. 2019. "Everything you need to know about omega 3". https://lifespa.com/omega-3-secret-unveiled-heart-brain-and-gut-support

Harvard T.H. Chan. 2018. "Monounsaturated fat from plants, not animals, may lower heart disease risk". https://www.hsph.harvard.edu/news/features/monosaturated-fat-heart-disease-risk

Khan Academy Medicine. 2014. "Overview of fatty acid oxidation" *Youtube.* [Embedded Video]. https://www.youtube.com/watch?v=acA5iF1zrDl

Kresser, C. 2019. "How too much omega-6 and not enough omega-3 is making us sick". https://chriskresser.com/how-too-much-omega-6-and-not-enough-omega-3-is-making-us-sick

Kresser, C. 2019. "Why fish stomps flax as a source of omega-3". https://chriskresser.com/why-fish-stomps-flax-seeds-as-a-source-of-omega-3

Kresser, C. 2019. "Should you really be taking fish oil?". https://chriskresser.com/should-you-really-be-taking-fish-oil

Lands, B. 2014. "Dietary omega-3 and omega-6 fatty acids compete in producing tissue compositions and tissue responses". *Military Medicine* 179 (11S): 76-81. https://doi.org/10.7205/milmed-d-14-00149

Oregon State University. n.d. "Essential fatty acids". https://lpi.oregonstate.edu/mic/other-nutrients/essential-fatty-acids

Qian, F. et. al. 2016. "Metabolic Effects of Monounsaturated Fatty Acid–Enriched Diets Compared With Carbohydrate or Polyunsaturated Fatty Acid–Enriched Diets in Patients With Type 2 Diabetes: A Systematic Review and Meta-analysis of Randomized Controlled Trials". *Diabetes Care* 39 (8): 1448–1457. https://doi.org/10.2337/dc16-0513

Raederstorff, D., et. al. 2015. "Vitamin E function and requirements in relation to PUFA". *Br J Nutr* 114 (8): 1113-122. https://doi.org/10.1017/S000711451500272X

Robertson, R. 2020. "Omega-3-6-9 fatty acids: A complete overview". https://www.healthline.com/nutrition/omega-3-6-9-overview

Simopoulos, A. P. 2016. "An increase in the omega-6/omega-3 fatty acid ratio increases the risk for obesity". *Nutrients* 8 (3): 128. https://doi.org/10.3390/nu8030128

## TRANS-FAT

Bridges, M. 2020. "Facts about trans fats". https://medlineplus.gov/ency/patientinstructions/000786.htm

Wu, J. , et. al. 2017. *Levels of trans fats in the food supply and consumption in Australia.* Expert Commentary brokered by the Sax Institute for The National. https://www.saxinstitute.org.au/wp-content/uploads/Expert-Commentary-Levels-of-trans-fats-in-the-food-supply-and-consumption-in-Australia.pdf

## DIETARY FIBRE

Australian Government. 2019. "Dietary fibre". National Health and Medical research council. https://www.nrv.gov.au/nutrients/dietary-fibre

Ballantyne, S. 2013. *The Paleo Approach: Reverse Autoimmune Disease and Heal Your Body.* Las Vegas: Victory Belt Publishing Inc. ISBN 978-1-936608-39-3

Bulsiewicz, W. 2020. *Fiber Fueled. The Plant-Based Gut Health Program for Losing Weight, Restoring Health, and Optimizing Your Microbiome.* Avery - an imprint of Penguin Random House, New York. [Kindle] ISBN 978059084571

Carlson, J. L., et. al. 2018. "Health effects and sources of prebiotic dietary fiber". *Curr Dev Nutr* 2 (3): nzy005. https://doi.org/10.1093/cdn/nzy005

Cholesterol and Fat Database. 2019. "Total dietary, soluble and insoluble fiber content of foods: Vegetables, fruits and legumes". https://www.dietaryfiberfood.com/dietary-fiber/fiber-content.php

Christensen, L. 2020. "The many types of fiber: Your guide to dietary fiber, prebiotics, and starches". https://chriskresser.com/types-of-dietary-fiber

Dietary Fiber Food. 2019. "Total dietary, soluble and insoluble fiber content of foods: Vegetables, fruits and legumes". https://www.dietaryfiberfood.com/dietary-fiber/fiber-content.php

El-Salhy, M., et. al. 2017. "Dietary fiber in Irritable Bowel Syndrome (Review)". *Int J Mol Med* 40 (3): 607-613. https://doi.org/10.3892/ijmm.2017.3072

Everyday Health. 2019. "Why is fiber important for your digestive health?" https://www.everydayhealth.com/digestive-health/experts-why-is-fiber-important.aspx

Higdon, J., et. al. 2019. "Fiber". Linus Pauling Institute. https://lpi.oregonstate.edu/mic/other-nutrients/fiber

Lambeau, K. V., et. al. 2017. "Fiber supplements and clinically proven health benefits: How to recognize and recommend an effective fiber therapy". *J Am Assoc Nurse Pract* 29 (4): 216-223. https://doi.org/10.1002/2327-6924.12447

Lattimer, J. M., et. al. 2010. "Effects of dietary fiber and its components on metabolic health". *Nutrients* 2 (12): 1266-89. https://doi.org/10.3390/nu2121266

Mayo Clinic staff. "Diverticulitis". Mayo Foundation. https://www.mayoclinic.org/diseases-conditions/diverticulitis/symptoms-causes/syc-20371758

McRorie, J. W., Jr. 2015. "Evidence-based approach to fiber supplements and clinically meaningful health benefits, part 2: What to look for and how to recommend an effective fiber therapy". Nutr Today 50 (2): 90-97. https://doi.org/10.1097/NT.0000000000000089

Shammas, M. A. 2011. "Telomeres, lifestyle, cancer, and aging". *Curr Opin Clin Nutr Metab Care* 14 (1): 28-34. https://doi.org/10.1097/MCO. 0b013e32834121b1

WebMD. n.d. "Types of fiber and their health benefits". https://www.webmd.com/diet/compare-dietary-fibers

## INSOLUBLE FIBRE

Ballantyne, S. 2015. "Resistant starch: It's not all sunshine and roses". https://www.thepaleomom. com/resistant-starch-its-not-all-sunshine-and-roses

Chung, W. S. F., et. al., 2017. "Prebiotic potential of pectin and pectic oligosaccharides to promote anti-inflammatory commensal bacteria in the human colon". *FEMS Microbiology Ecology* 93 (11). https://doi.org/10.1093/femsec/fix127

Cory, H., et. al. 2018. "The role of polyphenols in human health and food systems: A mini-review". *Front Nutr* 5: 87. https://doi.org/10.3389/ fnut.2018.00087

Edwards, C. A., et. al. 2017. "Polyphenols and health: Interactions between fibre, plant polyphenols and the gut microbiota". *Wiley, Nutrition Bulletin* 42 (4): 356-360. https://doi.org/10.1111/nbu.12296

Environmental Working Group. 2021. "Ewg's 2021 shopper's guide to pesticides in produce". https:// www.ewg.org/foodnews/dirty-dozen.php

Hassan, A. K., et. al. 2015. "An overview of fruit allergy and the causative allergens". *Eur Ann Allergy Clin Immunol* 47 (6): 180-7. https://www.ncbi.nlm.nih. gov/pubmed/26549334

Jakobek, L., et. al. 2019. "Non-covalent dietary fiber - Polyphenol interactions and their influence on polyphenol bioaccessibility". *Trends in Food Science & Technology* 83: 235-247. https://doi.org/10.1016/ j.tifs.2018.11.024

Jiang, T., et. al. 2016. "Apple-derived pectin modulates gut microbiota, improves gut barrier function, and attenuates metabolic endotoxemia in rats with diet-induced obesity". *Nutrients* 8 (3): 126. https:// doi.org/10.3390/nu8030126

Kamiya, T., et. al. 2014. "Therapeutic effects of biobran, modified arabinoxylan rice bran, in improving symptoms of diarrhea predominant or mixed type Irritable Bowel Syndrome: a pilot, randomized controlled study". *Evid Based Complement Alternat Med* 2014: 828137. https://doi.org/10.1155/2014/828137

Koutsos, A., et. al. 2015. "Apples and cardiovascular health--is the gut microbiota a core consideration?" *Nutrients* 7 (6): 3959-98. https://doi.org/10.3390/ nu7063959

Park, A. 2018. "Strawberries top the 'dirty dozen' list of fruits and vegetables with the most pesticides". Health Diet & Nutrition. Time, USA. https://time. com/5234787/dirty-dozen-pesticides

Scheller, H. V., et. al. 2010. "Hemicelluloses". *Annu Rev Plant Biol* 61: 263-89. https://doi.org/10.1146/ annurev-arplant-042809-112315

Speer, H., et. al. 2019. "The effects of dietary polyphenols on circulating cardiovascular disease biomarkers and iron status: A systematic review". *Nutr Metab Insights* 12: 1178638819882739. https:// doi.org/10.1177/1178638819882739

Timm, D. A., et. al. 2010. "Wheat dextrin, psyllium, and inulin produce distinct fermentation patterns, gas volumes, and short-chain fatty acid profiles in vitro". *J Med Food* 13 (4): 961-6. https://doi.org/ 10.1089/jmf.2009.0135

Varney, J. 2016. "Dietary fibre series - insoluble fibre". Monash University, Australia. Monash FODMAP blog. https://www.monashfodmap.com/blog/ dietary-fibre-series-insoluble-fibre

WebMD. n.d. "Arabinoxylan". https://www.webmd. com/vitamins/ai/ingredientmono-1455/ arabinoxylan

Wrong, Cathy. 2021. "The health benefits of arabinoxylan". https://www.verywellhealth.com/ the-benefits-of-arabinoxylan-89600

Xu, L., et. al. 2015. "Efficacy of pectin in the treatment of diarrhea predominant Irritable Bowel Syndrome". *Zhonghua Wei Chang Wai Ke Za Zhi* 18 (3): 267-71. https://www.ncbi.nlm.nih.gov/pubmed/25809332

## SOLUBLE FIBRE

Babiker, R., et. al. 2012. "Effects of Gum Arabic ingestion on body mass index and body fat percentage in healthy adult females: two-arm randomized, placebo controlled, double-blind trial". *Nutr J* 11: 111. https://doi.org/10.1186/1475-2891-11-111

Bashir, K. M., et. al. 2017. "Clinical and physiological perspectives of beta-glucans: The past, present, and future". *Int J Mol Sci* 18 (9). https://doi.org/10.3390/ ijms18091906

Butt, M.S., et. al., 2007. "Guar Gum: A Miracle Therapy for Hypercholesterolemia, Hyperglycemia and Obesity". *Critical Reviews in Food Science and Nutrition* 47 (4): 389-96. https://doi.org/ 10.1080/10408390600846267

Carter, A. 2019. "The health benefits of psyllium". https://www.healthline.com/health/psyllium-health-benefits

Chan, G. C.-F., et. al. 2009. "The effects of β-glucan on human immune and cancer cells". *Journal of Hematology & Oncology* 2 (1). https://doi.org/ 10.1186/1756-8722-2-25

Chawla, R., et. al. 2010. "Soluble dietary fiber". *Comprehensive Reviews in Food Science and Food Safety* 9 (2): 178-196. https://doi.org/ 10.1111/j.1541-4337.2009.00099.x

dos Santos Ourique Figueiredo, M., et. al. 2006. "Effect of guar gum supplementation on lipidic and glycidic metabolic control and body mass index in type 2 diabetes". *Review of Nutrition* 19 (2). https://doi.org/10.1590/S1415-52732006000200006

Daly, J., et. al. 1993. "The effect of feeding xanthan gum on colonic function in man: correlation with in vitro determinants of bacterial breakdown". *Br J Nutr* 69 (3): 897-902. https://doi.org/10.1079/bjn19930089

den Besten, G., et. al. 2013. "The role of short-chain fatty acids in the interplay between diet, gut microbiota, and host energy metabolism". *J Lipid Res.* 54 (9): 2325–2340. https://doi.org/10.1194/jlr.R036012

Donovan, P. 2007. "Inulin: Friend or foe?". https://www.naturalnews.com/022356_inulin_food_ingredients.html

El-Salhy, M., et. al. 2017. "Dietary fiber in Irritable Bowel Syndrome (Review)". *Int J Mol Med* 40 (3): 607-613. https://doi.org/10.3892/ijmm.2017.3072

Eltayeb, I. B. 2004. "Effect of Gum Arabic on the absorption of a single oral dose of amoxicillin in healthy Sudanese volunteers". *Journal of Antimicrobial Chemotherapy* 54 (2): 577-578. https://doi.org/10.1093/jac/dkh372

Giannini, E. G., et. al. 2006. "Role of partially hydrolyzed guar gum in the treatment of Irritable Bowel Syndrome". *Nutrition* 22 (3): 334-42. https://doi.org/10.1016/j.nut.2005.10.003

Haskey, N., et. al. 2017. "An Examination of Diet for the Maintenance of Remission in Inflammatory Bowel Disease". Nutrients 9 (3): 259. https://doi.org/10.3390/nu9030259

Kresser, C. 2017. "Harmful or Harmless: Xanthan Gum". https://chriskresser.com/harmful-or-harmless-xanthan-gum

Kresser, C. 2019. "Harmful or Harmless: Guar Gum, Locust Bean Gum, and More". https://chriskresser.com/harmful-or-harmless-guar-gum-locust-bean-gum-and-more

Lambeau, K. V., et. al. 2017. "Fiber supplements and clinically proven health benefits: How to recognize and recommend an effective fiber therapy". *J Am Assoc Nurse Pract* 29 (4): 216-223. https://doi.org/10.1002/2327-6924.12447

Pole, Sebastian. 2013. *Ayurvedic Medicine. The Principles of Traditional Practice*, Singing Dragon, London and Philadelphia. p. 160. ISBN 978-1-84819-113-6

Rideout, T. C., et. al. 2008. "Guar gum and similar soluble fibers in the regulation of cholesterol metabolism: current understandings and future research priorities". *Vasc Health Risk Manag* 4 (5): 1023-33. https://doi.org/10.2147/vhrm.s3512

Russo, L., et. al. 2015. "Partially hydrolyzed guar gum in the treatment of Irritable Bowel Syndrome with constipation: effects of gender, age, and body mass index". *Saudi J Gastroenterol* 21 (2): 104-10. https://doi.org/10.4103/1319-3767.153835

Timm, D. A., et. al. 2010. "Wheat dextrin, psyllium, and inulin produce distinct fermentation patterns, gas volumes, and short-chain fatty acid profiles in vitro". *J Med Food* 13 (4): 961-6. https://doi.org/10.1089/jmf.2009.0135

Wrong. C., et. al. 2016. "Potential Benefits of Dietary Fibre Intervention in Inflammatory Bowel Disease". *International Journal of Molecular Science* 17 (6): 919. https://doi.org/10.3390/ijms17060919

## BUTYRATE

Canani, R. B. 2011. "Potential beneficial effects of butyrate in intestinal and extraintestinal diseases". *World Journal of Gastroenterology* 17 (12). https://doi.org/10.3748/wjg.v17.i12.1519

Eyvazzadeh, A. 2019. "What is butyric acid, and does it have health benefits?". https://www.healthline.com/health/butyric-acid

Gill, R. K., et. al. 2011. "A novel facet to consider for the effects of butyrate on its target cells. Focus on "The short-chain fatty acid butyrate is a substrate of breast cancer resistance protein"". *American Journal of Physiology-Cell Physiology* 301 (5): C977-C979. https://doi.org/10.1152/ajpcell.00290.2011

Liu, H., et. al. "Butyrate: A double-edged sword for health?" *Advances in Nutrition* 9 (1): 21-29. https://doi.org/10.1093/advances/nmx009

Nigh, G. 2017. "Sulfur metabolism demystified and an alternative view of SIBO". Interview by Shivan Sarna. *SIBO SOS Summit*. [Transcript]. Chronic Condition Rescue. https://sibosos.com/summits

Nigh, G. 2017. "Supplements & treatments to increase Sulfur Metabolism". Interview by Shivan Sarna. *SIBO SOS Summit*. [transcript]. Chronic Condition Rescue. https://sibosos.com/summits

Scheppach, W., et. al., 1992. "Effect of butyrate enemas on the colonic mucosa in distal ulcerative colitis". *Gastroenterology* 103 (1): 51-56. https://doi.org/10.1016/0016-5085(92)91094-k

Załęski, A., et. al. 2013. "Butyric acid in Irritable Bowel Syndrome". *Gastroenterology Review* 6: 350-353. https://doi.org/10.5114/pg.2013.39917

## DAIRY

ASCIA Committee and Working Party Members. 2020. "Dietary guide for food allergy". Australian Society of Clinical Immunology and Allery. https://www.allergy.org.au/images/pcc/ASCIA_PCC_Dietary_Avoidance_Cows_Milk_2020.pdf

Beyond Celiac. n.d. "Celiac disease and lactose intolerance". https://www.beyondceliac.org/celiac-disease/related-conditions/lactose-intolerance

Cafasso, J. 2021. "How to Tell the Difference Between IBS and Lactose Intolerance". https://www.healthline.com/health/ibs-vs-lactose-intolerance

Clemons, R. 2015. "Coconut drink recalls: cow's milk not declared on label". https://www.choice.com.au/food-and-drink/food-warnings-and-safety/food-safety/articles/coconut-drinks-with-dairy-allergens-recall-081015#table

College of Agriculture and Life Sciences Cornell University. n.d. "Milk facts". Department of Food and Science. http://www.milkfacts.info/Milk%20Composition/Carbohydrate.htm

Food and Agriculture Organisation of the United Nations. n.d. "Dairy animals". http://www.fao.org/dairy-production-products/production/dairy-animals/en

Frestedt, J. L., et. al. 2008. "A whey-protein supplement increases fat loss and spares lean muscle in obese subjects: a randomized human clinical study". *Nutr Metab (Lond)* 5: 8. https://doi.org/10.1186/1743-7075-5-8

Heins, B. 2021. "Grass-fed cows produce healthier milk". University of Minnesota. https://extension.umn.edu/pasture-based-dairy/grass-fed-cows-produce-healthier-milk

Jacob, A. 2018". Casein protein intolerance". https://healthyeating.sfgate.com/casein-protein-intolerance-2028.html

Ji, J., et. al. 2015. "Lactose intolerance and risk of lung, breast and ovarian cancers: aetiological clues from a population-based study in Sweden". *Br J Cancer* 112 (1): 149-52. https://doi.org/10.1038/bjc.2014.544

Kinman, T. 2020. "What Is a Lactose Tolerance Test?". https://www.healthline.com/health/lactose-tolerance-tests

Mayo Clinic staff. n.d. "Giardia infection (giardiasis)". Mayo Foundation. https://www.mayoclinic.org/diseases-conditions/giardia-infection/symptoms-causes/syc-20372786

McGregor, R. A., et. al. 2013. "Milk protein for improved metabolic health: a review of the evidence". *Nutr Metab (Lond)* 10 (1): 46. https://doi.org/10.1186/1743-7075-10-46

NSW Government. n.d. "Dientamoeba fragilis fact sheet". https://www.health.nsw.gov.au/Infectious/factsheets/Pages/dientamoeba-fragilis.aspx

Pal, S., et. al. 2015. "Milk Intolerance, Beta-Casein and Lactose". *Nutrients* 7 (9): 7285-97. https://doi.org/10.3390/nu7095339

Sodhi, M., et. al. 2012. "Milk proteins and human health: A1/A2 milk hypothesis". *Indian Journal of Endocrinology and Metabolism* 16 (5): 856. https://doi.org/10.4103/2230-8210.100685

## WHEY PROTEIN

Mayo Clinic staff. n.d. "Whey protein". Mayo Foundation. https://www.mayoclinic.org/drugs-supplements-whey-protein/art-20363344

Sugawara, K., et. al., 2012. "Effect of anti-inflammatory supplementation with whey peptide and exercise therapy in patients with COPD". *Respiratory Medicine* 106 (11): 1526-1534. https://doi.org/10.1016/j.rmed.2012.07.001

Tosukhowong, P., et. at. 2016. "Biochemical and clinical effects of Whey protein supplementation in Parkinson's disease: A pilot study". Journal of the Neurological Sciences 367:162-70. https://doi.org/10.1016/j.jns.2016.05.056

WebMD. n.d. "Whey protein". https://www.webmd.com/vitamins/ai/ingredientmono-833/whey-protein#main-container

## CAMEL MILK

Cardoso, R. R., et. al. 2010. "Consumption of camel's milk by patient's intolerant to lactose. A preliminary study". *Rev Alerg Mex* 57 (1): 26-32. https://www.ncbi.

nlm.nih.gov/pubmed/20857626

Salmen, S. H., et. al. 2012. "Amino acids content and electrophoretic profile of camel milk casein from different camel breeds in Saudi Arabia". *Saudi J Biol Sci* 19 (2): 177-83. https://doi.org/10.1016/j.sjbs.2011.12.002

Zibaee, S., et. al. 2015. "Nutritional and Therapeutic Characteristics of Camel Milk in Children: A Systematic Review". *Electron Physician* 7 (7): 1523-8. https://doi.org/10.19082/1523

## MARE'S MILK

Neal, B. 2018. "Horse milk is apparently a growing trend in Europe & here's why". https://www.bustle.com/p/what-is-mare-milk-horse-milk-is-apparently-a-growing-trend-in-europe-9842844

Nurtazin, S., et. al. 2016. "Mare's milk and kumys". Вестник КазНУ Серия Экологическая 43. https://www.researchgate.net/publication/303486997_Mare's_milk_and_kumys

Pieszka, M., et. al. 2016. "Is mare milk an appropriate food for people? – a review". *Annals of Animal Science* 16 (1): 33-51. https://doi.org/10.1515/aoas-2015-0041

## GHEE

Amidor, T. 2016. "Ask the expert: Ghee butter". https://www.todaysdietitian.com/newarchives/1016p10.shtml

Douillard, J. n.d. "Ghee 101". https://lifespa.com/ayurvedic-supplement-facts/ghee

Reddy, A., et. al. 2013. "Myths and facts about consumption of ghee in relation to heart problems - a comparative research study". International Journal of Pharmacy and Pharmaceutical Sciences. https://innovareacademics.in/journal/ijpps/Vol5Suppl2/6940.pdf

Sharma, H., et. al. 2010. "The effect of ghee (clarified butter) on serum lipid levels and microsomal lipid peroxidation". *Ayu* 31 (2): 134-40. https://doi.org/10.4103/0974-8520.72361

## GLUTEN

De Punder, K., et. al. 2013. "The dietary intake of wheat and other cereal grains and their role in inflammation". *Nutrients* 5 (3): 771-787. https://doi.org/10.3390/nu5030771

Fasano, A. 2011. "Zonulin and its regulation of intestinal barrier function: The biological door to inflammation, autoimmunity, and cancer". *Physiological Reviews* 91 (1): 151-175. https://doi.org/10.1152/physrev.00003.2008

## CELIAC DISEASE

Balakireva, A., et. al. 2016. "Properties of gluten intolerance: Gluten structure, evolution, pathogenicity and detoxification capabilities". *Nutrients* 8 (10). https://doi.org/10.3390/nu8100644

Barone, M., et. al. 2014. "Gliadin peptides as triggers of the proliferative and stress/innate immune response of the celiac small intestinal mucosa". *International Journal of Molecular Sciences* 15 (11): 20518-20537. https://doi.org/10.3390/ijms151120518

Béres, J. N., et. al. 2016. "Role of the microbiome in celiac disease". *International Journal of Celiac Disease* 2 (4): 150-153. https://doi.org/10.12691/ijcd-2-4-4

Bulsiewicz, W. 2020. *Fiber Fueled. The Plant-Based Gut Health Program for Losing Weight, Restoring Your Health, and Optimizing Your Microbiome.* Avery, an imprint of Pinguin Random House LLC, New York. [Kindle] ISBN 9780593084571

Cecilio, L. A., et. al. 2015. "The prevalence of Hla Dq2 and Dq8 in patients with celiac disease, in family and in general population". *ABCD. Arquivos Brasileiros de Cirurgia Digestiva (São Paulo)* 28 (3): 183-185. https://doi.org/10.1590/s0102-67202015000300009

Chander, A.M., 2018. "Cross-Talk Between Gluten, Intestinal Microbiota and Intestinal Mucosa in Celiac Disease: Recent Advances and Basis of Autoimmunity". *Frontiers Microbiology* 9: 2597. https://doi.org/10.3389/fmicb.2018.02597

Coeliac Australia. n.d. "Conditions associated with Coeliac Disease". https://www.coeliac.org.au/s/article/Associated-Conditions-CD

Coeliac Australia. n.d. "Coeliac Disease Brochure". https://www.coeliac.org.au/s/article/Coeliac-disease

Coeliac Australia. n.d. "Symptoms". https://www.coeliac.org.au/s/coeliac-disease/symptoms

Celiac Disease Foundation, n.d. "What is Celiac Disease?". https://celiac.org/about-celiac-disease/what-is-celiac-disease

Celiac Disease Foundation, 2014. "Gluten alternatives: Effects of eating quinoa in celiac patients". https://celiac.org/about-the-foundation/featured-news/2014/02/gluten-alternatives-effects-of-eating-quinoa-in-celiac-patients

Elli, L., et. al. 2015. "Diagnosis of gluten related disorders: Celiac disease, wheat allergy and non-celiac gluten sensitivity". *World J Gastroenterol* 21 (23): 7110-9. https://doi.org/10.3748/wjg.v21.i23.7110

Hollon, J., et. al. 2015. "Effect of gliadin on permeability of intestinal biopsy explants from celiac disease patients and patients with non-celiac gluten sensitivity". *Nutrients* 7 (3): 1565-1576. https://doi.org/10.3390/nu7031565

Kupfer, S. S. 2009. "Making sense of marsh". [PDF]. Celiac Disease Center of the University of Chicago. https://www.cureceliacdisease.org/wp-content/uploads/0909CeliacCtr_News_v3final.pdf

Marsh, M. N., et. al. 2015. "Mucosal histopathology in celiac disease: a rebuttal of Oberhuber's sub-division of Marsh III". *Gastroenterol Hepatol Bed Bench* 8 (2): 99-109. https://www.ncbi.nlm.nih.gov/pubmed/25926934

Rezania, K. 2010. "Celiac Neuropathy". [PDF]. Celiac Disease Center of the University of Chicago. https://www.cureceliacdisease.org/wp-content/uploads/0410CeliacCtr_News.pdf

Sapone, A., et. al., 2012. "Spectrum of gluten-related disorders: consensus on new nomenclature and classification". *BMC Medicine* 10 (1). https://doi.org/10.1186/1741-7015-10-13

Tursi, A., et. al. 2003. "High prevalence of Small Intestinal Bacterial Overgrowth in celiac patients with persistence of gastrointestinal symptoms after gluten withdrawal". *The American Journal of Gastroenterology* 98 (4): 839-843. https://doi.org/10.1111/j.1572-0241.2003.07379.x

Verdu, E. F., et. al. 2009. "Between celiac disease and Irritable Bowel Syndrome: the "no man's land" of gluten sensitivity". *Am J Gastroenterol* 104 (6): 1587-94. https://doi.org/10.1038/ajg.2009.188

Vojdani, A., et. al. 2013. "Cross-reaction between gliadin and different food and tissue antigens". *Food and Nutrition Sciences* 04 (01): 20-32. https://doi.org/10.4236/fns.2013.41005

Willoughby, D. S. 2014. "The role of the gluten-derived peptide gliadin in celiac disease". *Journal of Nutritional Health & Food Engineering* 1 (6). https://doi.org/10.15406/jnhfe.2014.01.00036

Wu, H., et. al. 2018. "Challenges with Point-Of-Care Tests (POCT) for Celiac Disease". *Celiac Disease - From the Bench to the Clinic.* https://doi.org/10.5772/intechopen.81874

Zanini, B., et. al., 2013. "Celiac disease with mild enteropathy is not mild disease". *Clinical Gastroenterology and Hepatology* 11 (3): 253-258. https://doi.org/10.1016/j.cgh.2012.09.027

## NON-CELIAC GLUTEN SENSITIVITY

Andrews, R. n.d. "All about lectins: Here's what you need to know". https://www.precisionnutrition.com/all-about-lectins

Bai, J. C., et. al., 2010. "New serology assays can detect gluten sensitivity among enteropathy patients seronegative for anti–tissue transglutaminase". *Clinical Chemistry* 56 (4): 661-665. https://doi.org/10.1373/clinchem.2009.129668

Balakireva, A., et. al. 2016. "Properties of gluten intolerance: Gluten structure, evolution, pathogenicity and detoxification capabilities". *Nutrients* 8 (10). https://doi.org/10.3390/nu8100644

Biesiekierski, J. R., et. al. 2013. "No effects of gluten in patients with self-reported non-celiac gluten sensitivity after dietary reduction of fermentable, poorly absorbed, short-chain carbohydrates". *Gastroenterology* 145 (2): 320-8.e1-3. https://doi.org/10.1053/j.gastro.2013.04.051

Bulka, C. M., et. al. 2017. "The unintended consequences of a gluten-free diet". *Epidemiology* 28 (3): e24-e25. https://doi.org/10.1097/EDE.0000000000000640

Cebolla, Á., et. al. 2018. "Gluten immunogenic peptides as standard for the evaluation of potential harmful prolamin content in food and human specimen". *Nutrients* 10 (12). https://doi.org/10.3390/nu10121927

Jones, A. L. 2017. "Jones, A. L. 2017. "The Gluten-Free Diet: Fad or Necessity?" Diabetes Spectrum 30 (2): 118-123. *Diabetes Spectrum* 30 (2): 118-123. https://doi.org/10.2337/ds16-0022

Makharia, A., et. al. 2015. "The overlap between Irritable Bowel Syndrome and non-celiac gluten sensitivity: A clinical dilemma". *Nutrients* 7 (12): 10417-26. https://doi.org/10.3390/nu7125541

Elli, L., et. al. 2015. "Diagnosis of gluten related disorders: Celiac disease, wheat allergy and non-celiac gluten sensitivity". *World J Gastroenterol* 21 (23): 7110-9. https://doi.org/10.3748/wjg.v21.i23.7110

Hollon, J., et. al. 2015. "Effect of gliadin on permeability of intestinal biopsy explants from celiac disease patients and patients with non-celiac gluten sensitivity". *Nutrients* 7 (3): 1565-1576. https://doi.org/10.3390/nu7031565

Sapone, A., et. al. 2012. "Spectrum of gluten-related disorders: consensus on new nomenclature and classification". *BMC Medicine* 10 (1). https://doi.org/10.1186/1741-7015-10-13

## A WORD ON OATS

Balakireva, A., et. al. 2016. "Properties of gluten intolerance: Gluten structure, evolution, pathogenicity and detoxification capabilities". *Nutrients* 8 (10). https://doi.org/10.3390/nu8100644

Bjarnadottir, A., 2019. "Oats 101: Nutrition Facts and Health Benefits". https://www.healthline.com/nutrition/foods/oats

Cebolla, Á., et. al. 2018. "Gluten immunogenic peptides as standard for the evaluation of potential harmful prolamin content in food and human specimen". *Nutrients* 10 (12). https://doi.org/10.3390/nu10121927

Comino, I., et. al. 2015. "Role of oats in celiac disease". *World J Gastroenterol* 21 (41): 11825-31. https://doi.org/10.3748/wjg.v21.i41.11825

Gluten and Allery Free Passport. n.d. "Food labelling by region". https://glutenfreepassport.com/pages/understand-global-gluten-free-amp-food-allergy-product-labeling

Gluten Free Oats. n.d. "Gluten-free labelling laws in Australia around Oats". https://gfoats.com.au/gluten-free-labelling-laws-in-australia-around-oats-Coeliac Australia. 2015. "Oats and the gluten free diet". https://www.coeliac.org.au/s/article/Oats-and-the-gluten-free-diet

Celiac Disease Foundation. 2016. "NASSCD Releases Summary Statement on Oats". https://celiac.org/about-the-foundation/featured-news/2016/04/nasscd-releases-summary-statement-on-oats

Mäkinen, O.E., et. al. 2016. "Protein From Oat: Structure, Processes, Functionality, and Nutrition". Academic Press, *Sustainable Protein Sources* (6): 105-119. https://doi.org/10.1016/B978-0-12-802778-3.00006-8

## DIETS

Kinney, K. 2015. "Why Diet alone is not enough to treat SIBO". https://chriskresser.com/why-diet-alone-is-not-enough-to-treat-sibo

Sapone, A., et. al., 2012. "Spectrum of gluten-related disorders: consensus on new nomenclature and classification". *BMC Medicine* 10 (1). https://doi.org/10.1186/1741-7015-10-13

Spiegel. 2021. "Menschen ernähren sich heute weniger vielfältig als vor 100 Jahren". https://www.spiegel.

de/wissenschaft/mensch/ernaehrung-menschen-essen-heute-weniger-vielfaeltig-als-vor-100-jahren-a-382ed207-63ec-4dc9-88d4-da69b4fe46dc

Bird, M. I., et. al. 2021. "A global carbon and nitrogen isotope perspective on modern and ancient human diet". *Proc Natl Acad Sci U S A* 118 (19). https://doi.org/10.1073/pnas.2024642118

## SPECIFIC CARBOHYDRATE DIET

Cohen, S. A., et. al. 2014. "Clinical and mucosal improvement with specific carbohydrate diet in pediatric Crohn disease". *J Pediatr Gastroenterol Nutr* 59 (4): 516-21. https://doi.org/10.1097/MPG.0000000000000449

Dubrovsky, A., et. al. 2018. "Effect of the Specific Carbohydrate Diet on the Microbiome of a Primary Sclerosing Cholangitis and Ulcerative Colitis Patient". *Cureus* 10 (2): e2177. https://doi.org/10.7759/cureus.2177

Guandalini, S. 2007. "A brief history of celiac disease". Celiac Disease Center of the University of Chicago. [PDF]. http://www.cureceliacdisease.org/wp-content/uploads/SU07CeliacCtr.News_.pdf

Mueller, K. 2016. "Novel diet therapy helps children with Crohn's disease and Ulcerative Colitis reach remission". Seattle Children's Hospital. Gastroenterology. https://pulse.seattlechildrens.org/novel-diet-therapy-helps-children-with-crohns-disease-and-ulcerative-colitis-reach-remission

Obih, C., et. al. 2016. "Specific carbohydrate diet for pediatric inflammatory bowel disease in clinical practice within an academic IBD center". *Nutrition* 32 (4): 418-25. https://doi.org/10.1016/j.nut.2015.08.025

SCDiet. 2000. "About Dr. Sydney Valentine Haas". https://www.scdiet.net/scdarchive/1about/haas-biblio.html

SCD Diet. n.d. "Breaking the Vicious Cycle. Intestinal health through diet with the specific carbohydrate diet". http://www.breakingtheviciouscycle.info

Sherwood, A. 2020. "What is the specific carbohydrate diet?". https://www.webmd.com/ibd-crohns-disease/crohns-disease/specific-carbohydrate-diet-overview#1

Suskind, D. L., et. al. 2016. "Patients perceive clinical benefit with the specific carbohydrate diet for inflammatory bowel disease". *Dig Dis Sci* 61 (11): 3255-3260. https://doi.org/10.1007/s10620-016-4307-y

Wikipedia Encyclopedia. n.d. "Sidney V. Haas". https://en.wikipedia.org/wiki/Sidney_V._Haas

## LOW-FODMAP DIET

Farmer, J. 2018. "Why garlic is so bad for IBS and diarrhoea symptoms". https://www.telegraph.co.uk/food-and-drink/fodmap-advice-and-recipes/why-garlic-makes-ibs-worse

Gibson, P. R., et. al. 2010. "Evidence-based dietary management of functional gastrointestinal symptoms: The FODMAP approach". *Journal of Gastroenterology and Hepatology* 25 (2): 252-258. https://doi.org/10.1111/j.1440-1746.2009.06149.x

Monash FODMAP team. 2015. "Cooking with onion and garlic - myths and facts". Monash University, FODMAP blog. https://www.monashfodmap.com/blog/cooking-with-onion-and-garlic-myths-and

Monash University. "The Low FODMAP Diet". https://www.monashfodmap.com

Varney, J. 2015. "The Monash University Low FODMAP Diet™ – NOT a 'lifetime' diet". Monash University Australia, FODMAP blog. https://www.monashfodmap.com/blog/low-fodmap-diet-not-lifetime-diet

## SIBO SPECIFIC FOOD GUIDE

Siebecker, A. 2014. "SIBO Specific food guide". [PDF]. https://www.siboinfo.com/uploads/5/4/8/4/5484269/sibo_specific_food_guide_nov_5_2014.pdf

## GUT AND PSYCHOLOGY DIET

Campbell-McBride, N. 2010. "Welcome to my site!". http://www.doctor-natasha.com

Campbell-McBride, N. 2016. "Interview: Dr. Natasha Campbell-McBride discusses the science behind gaps, modern nutrition woes". Interview by Tracy Frisch. https://www.ecofarmingdaily.com/interview-natasha-campbell-mcbride-on-gut-health

GAPS Diet Australia. 2011. "GAPS protocol". https://gapsaustralia.com.au/gaps-protocol

GAPS Diet Australia. 2018. "What is GAPS?". https://www.gapsdiet.com/about

Gillan, K. 2016. "GAPS diet: Do its claims to heal leaky gut and treat autism stand up?". https://coach.nine.com.au/diet/gaps-diet/6069962c-be87-42e7-bde8-06621d1eaa76

Weil, A. 2013. "GAPS Diet: How good is it?". https://www.drweil.com/diet-nutrition/diets-weight-loss/gaps-diet-how-good-is-it

## CEDARS-SINAI DIET

Siebecker, A. n.d. "Cedars-Sinai Diet (C-SD)". Cedars Sinai. [PDF]. https://www.siboinfo.com/uploads/5/4/8/4/5484269/low_fermentation_diet.pdf

## SIBO BI-PHASIC DIET

Carnahan, J. 2012. "Herxheimer reactions and die-off: Causes, symptoms, and preventing overgrowth". https://www.jillcarnahan.com/2012/11/17/tips-for-dealing-with-herxheimer-or-die-off-reactions

Jacobi, N. 2016. "The Sibo Bi-Phasic Diet, testing and herbal treatments with Dr. Nirala Jacobi," Interview by Rebecca Coomes. The Healthy Gut Podcast Ep. 4. [Audio]. https://thehealthygut.com/podcast/herbaltreatments

Jacobi, N. 2017. "SIBO SOS Summit". Interview by Shivan Sarna. SIBO SOS Summit. [Transcript]. Chronic Condition Rescue. https://sibosos.com/summits

Jacobi, N. 2019. "Launching the vegetarian SIBO Bi-Phasic diet". Facebook. [Embedded Video]. https://www.facebook.com/thesibodoctor/videos/311189252884384

The SIBO Doctor. n.d. "Get started with Dr Jacobi's Bi-Phasic approach". [PDF]. https://www.thesibodoctor.com/sibo-bi-phasic-diet-free-downloads

## FAST TRACT DIET

Robillard, N. 2013. Fast tract digestion IBS. First edition. Self Health Publishing, USA. [Kindle] ISBN 978-0-9766425-2-7

Robillard, N. 2017. "Choosing diet over drugs". Interview by Shivan Sarna. SIBO SOS Summit. [Transcript] ChronicCondition Rescue. https://sibo-sos.com/summits

Tanaka, R. 2014. "What foods can lead to SIBO? Try FP calculator". https://digestivehealthinstitute.org/2014/06/30/sibo-fp-calculator

## ELEMENTAL DIET

Altman, L. 2017. "The Elemental Diet for SIBO and other gut conditions". Interview by Tina Kaczor. [Transcript]. https://www.naturalmedicinejournal.com/journal/2017-09/elemental-diet-sibo-and-other-gut-conditions

Coomes, R. 2018. "The elemental diet with Rebecca Coomes Ep. 74". The healthy gut podcast. [Audio]. https://thehealthygut.com/podcast/elemental-diet

Kinney, K. 2019. "Can a Short-Term Elemental Diet Help Treat SIBO?". https://chriskresser.com/can-a-short-term-elemental-diet-help-treat-sibo

Koretz, R. L., et. al. 1980. "Elemental diets—Facts and fantasies". Gastroenterology 78 (2): 393-410. https://doi.org/10.1016/0016-5085(80)90594-6

Pimentel, M., et. al. 2004. "A 14-day elemental diet is highly effective in normalizing the lactulose breath test". Dig Dis Sci 49 (1): 73-7. https://doi.org/10.1023/b:ddas.0000011605.43979.e1

Rostami, K., et. al. 2015. "Elemental diets role in treatment of high ileostomy output and other gastrointestinal disorders". Gastroenterol Hepatol Bed Bench 8 (1): 71-6. https://www.ncbi.nlm.nih.gov/pubmed/25584179

Ruscio, M. 2018. Healthy Gut, Healthy You. A Personalized Plan to Transform Your Health from the Inside Out. The Ruscio Institute, Las Vegas. [Kindle] ISBN 978099766811

Ruscio, M. 2018. "Diving into the Elemental Diet (and mixing some up)". Interview by Shivan Sarna. https://drruscio.com/diving-into-the-elemental-diet

Sabourin, J. 2018. "The ultimate elemental diet guide for SIBO". https://sibosurvivor.com/elemental-diet-for-sibo

## NUTRITIONAL STRATEGY

ImuPro. 2016. "ImuPro", accompanying patient material, german [Paper].

ImuPro. n.d. "Professional guidance: Your nutritional strategy". https://imupro.com/your-imupro/nutritional-strategy

## AUTOIMMUNE PALEO DIET

Ballantyne, S. 2012. "The whys behind the Autoimmune Protocol: Nightshades". https://www.thepaleomom.com/the-whys-behind-autoimmune-protocol

Ballantyne, S. 2013. The Paleo Approach: Reverse Autoimmune Disease and Heal Your Body. Las Vegas: Victory Belt Publishing Inc. p. 140 – 185.

ISBN978-1-936608-39-3

Beth Schoenfeld, L. 2019 "AIP diet: What it is and specific steps for personalizing it for best health results". https://chriskresser.com/5-steps-to-personalizing-your-autoimmune-paleo-protocol

Jacob, A. 2013. "Gut health and autoimmune disease — Research suggests digestive abnormalities may be the underlying cause". https://www.todaysdietitian.com/newarchives/021313p38.shtml

Konijeti, G. G., et. al., 2017. "Efficacy of the autoimmune protocol diet for inflammatory bowel disease". *Inflamm Bowel Dis* 23 (11): 2054-2060. https://doi.org/10.1097/MIB.0000000000001221

Opazo, M. C., et. al., 2018. "Intestinal microbiota influences non-intestinal related autoimmune diseases". *Front Microbiol* 9: 432. https://doi.org/10.3389/fmicb.2018.00432

## WHOLE 30 DIET

Hartwig, D., et. al. *The Whole30*. 2015. Great Britain: Yellow Kite, imprint of Hodder & Stoughton, London. [Kindle] ISBN 978 1 473 61954 8.

Whole30. 2018. "The official Whole30 program rules". [PDF]. https://drruscio.com/wp-content/uploads/2018/09/official-whole30-program-rules.pdf

## THE MEDITERRANEAN STYLE DIET

Del Chierico, F., et. al. 2014. "Mediterranean Diet and Health: Food Effects on Gut Microbiota and Disease Control". *Int J Mol Sci* 15 (7): 11678–11699. https://doi.org/10.3390/ijms150711678

The fast 800. n. d. "Our Approaches". https://thefast800.com/the-very-fast-800

Tisgalou, C., et. al. 2021. "Gut microbiome and Mediterranean diet in the context of obesity. Current knowledge, perspectives and potential therapeutic targets". *Metabolism Open* Vol 9. https://doi.org/10.1016/j.metop.2021.100081

Varney, J. 2016. "A low FODMAP Mediterranean-style diet". https://www.monashfodmap.com/blog/a-low-fodmap-mediterranean-style-diet

Ventriglio, A., et. al. 2020. "Mediterranean Diet and its Benefits on Health and Mental Health: A Literature Review. *Clin Pract Epidemiol Ment Health* 16 (Suppl-1): 156–164. https://doi.org/10.2174/1745017902016010156

Zito, F. P., et. al. 2016. "Good adherence to mediterranean diet can prevent gastrointestinal symptoms: A survey from Southern Italy". *World J Gastrointest Pharmacol Ther.* 7 (4): 564–571. https://doi.org/10.4292/wjgpt.v7.i4.564

## AYURVEDA

Banyan Botanicals. n.d. "Ayurvedic food combining". https://www.banyanbotanicals.com/info/ayurvedic-living/living-ayurveda/diet/ayurvedic-food-combining

Johns Hopkins Medicine. 2020. "What is Ayurveda?" The John Hopkins University. https://www.hopkinsmedicine.org/health/wellness-and-prevention/ayurveda

Lad, U., et. al. n.d. "Incompatible food combining". The Ayurvedic Institute. https://www.ayurveda.com/resources/food-and-nutrition/incompatible-food-combining

Marshall, N. 2021. "About Ayurveda". Mudita Institute & Health Clinic, Australia. https://www.muditainstitute.com

Marshall, N. 2021. "Food Freedom with Ayurveda - Online course" [Video]. http://foodfreedomwithayurveda.com

Narayanaswamy, V. 1981. "Origin and development of Ayurveda (a brief history)". [PDF]. Ancient Science of Life. https://www.ncbi.nlm.nih.gov/pmc/articles/PMC3336651/pdf/ASL-1-1.pdf

Pattathu, A. G. 2018. "Ayurveda and discursive formations between Religion, Medicine and Embodiment". In *Medicine - Religion - Spirituality*, 133-166. ISBN: 9783839445822. Doi: 10.14361/9783839445822-006

Ramaswamy, S. 2018. "6 Superstar Spices of Ayurveda, plus 3 Recipes". https://chopra.com/articles/6-superstar-spices-of-ayurveda-plus-3-recipes

World Health Organization. 2013. *WHO Traditional Medicine Strategy 2014-2023*. WHO Library Cataloguing-in-Publication Data. https://www.who.int/publications/i/item/9789241506096

## SEASONAL EATING

Andrews, K., et. al. 2019. "Insect Population and Species decline a 'Wake-Up Call', Scientists say". *ABC Science*. ABC News, Australia. https://www.abc.net.au/news/science/2019-02-12/insect-species-in-decline-and-facing-extinction/10804094

Carey, T. 2017. "Gut microbes found in hunter-gatherers shift with the seasons". PBS News Hour. https://www.pbs.org/newshour/science/gut-microbes-found-hunter-gatherers-shift-seasons

Douillard, J. 2020. "Stanford study backs seasonal eating for the healthiest microbiome". https://lifespa.com/stanford-study-backs-seasonal-eating-for-healthiest-microbiome

Macdiarmid, J. I. 2013. "Seasonality and dietary requirements: will eating seasonal food contribute to health and environmental sustainability?" *Proceedings of the Nutrition Society* 73 (3): 368-375. https://doi.org/10.1017/s0029665113003753

Price, M. 2017. "Early human gut bacteria may have cycled with the season". American Association for Advancement of Science. https://www.sciencemag.org/news/2017/08/early-human-gut-bacteria-may-have-cycled-season

Sánchez-Bayo, F., et. al. 2019. "Worldwide decline of the entomofauna: A review of its drivers". *Biological Conservation* 232: 8-27. https://doi.org/10.1016/j.biocon.2019.01.020

Smith, C. 2019. "Insect Armageddon? Study shows 'catastrophic' declines in bug numbers," *The Science Show*. ABC Radio National. https://www.abc.net.au/radionational/programs/scienceshow/review-shows-catastrophic-declines-in-bug-numbers/10807270

Smits, S. A., et. al., 2017. "Seasonal cycling in the gut microbiome of the Hadza hunter-gatherers of Tanzania". *Science* 357 (6353): 802-806. https://doi.org/10.1126/science.aan4834

The art of eating

Cagampang, F. R., et. al. 2012. "The role of the circadian clock system in nutrition and metabolism". *British Journal of Nutrition*, 108 (3): 381 – 392. https://doi.org/10.1017/S0007114512002139

Codoner-Franch, P., et. al. 2018. "Circadian rhythms in the pathogenesis of gastrointestinal diseases". *World J Gastroenterol* 24 (38): 4297-4303. https://doi.org/10.3748/wjg.v24.i38.4297

David, M. 2005. *The Slow Down Diet: Eating for Pleasure, Energy, and Weight Loss*. Healing Arts Press, Vermont US. [Kindle] ISBN 978-1-62055-509-5

Davis, N. 2017. "Nobel Prize for Medicine awarded for Insights into Internal Biological Clock". http://www.theguardian.com/science/2017/oct/02/nobel-prize-for-medicine-awarded-for-insights-into-internal-biological-clock

Fuhrman, J. 2017. "ANDI Food Scores: Rating the Nutrient Density of Foods". https://www.drfuhrman.com/blog/128/andi-food-scores-rating-the-nutrient-density-of-foods

Harvard T.H. Chan. n.d. "The best Diet: Quality counts". School of Public Health. https://www.hsph.harvard.edu/nutritionsource/healthy-weight/best-diet-quality-counts

Konturek, P. C., et. al. 2011. "Gut clock: implication of circadian rhythms in the gastrointestinal tract". *J Physiol Pharmacol* 62 (2): 139-50. https://www.ncbi.nlm.nih.gov/pubmed/21673361

Laursen, M. 2017. "Ayurveda and Cycles of Time: How the Doshas Rule the Day". California Collages of Ayurveda. https://www.ayurvedacollege.com/blog/ayurveda-and-cycles-time-how-doshas-rule-day

Lopez-Minguez, J., et. al. 2019. "Timing of breakfast, lunch, and dinner. Effects on obesity and metabolic risk". Nutrients 11 (11). https://doi.org/10.3390/nu11112624

Manoogian, E. N. C., et. al. 2019. "When to Eat: The Importance of Eating Patterns in Health and Disease". *Journal of Biological Rhythms* 34 (6): 579-581. https://doi.org/10.1177/0748730419892105

National Institute of General Medical Sciences. n.d. "Circadian Rhythms". https://www.nigms.nih.gov/education/fact-sheets/Pages/circadian-rhythms.aspx

Newth, D., et. al. 2015. "Uncovering the Nutritional Landscape of Food". *Plos One* 10 (3). https://doi.org/10.1371/journal.pone.0118697

Nobel Foundation. 2017. "2017 Nobel Prize in Physiology or Medicine: Molecular mechanisms controlling the Circadian Rhythm. https://www.sciencedaily.com/releases/2017/10/171002092603.htm

Paoli, A., et. al. 2019. "The influence of meal frequency and timing on health in humans: The role of fasting". *Nutrients* 11 (4). https://doi.org/10.3390/nu11040719

Vaughn, B., et. al. 2014. "Circadian rhythm and sleep influences on digestive physiology and disorders". *ChronoPhysiology and Therapy*. https://doi.org/10.2147/cpt.S44806

**PERSONAL BOXES**

Asprey, D. n.d. "What Dr. Mercola didn't say about Dark Chocolate and Cardiovascular Disease". https://daveasprey.com/what-dr-mercola-didnt-say-about-dark-chocolate-and-cardiovascular-disease

Bode, A. M., et. al. "The Amazing and Mighty Ginger". In *Herbal Medicine: Biomolecular and Clinical Aspects*. Boca Raton (FL). https://www.ncbi.nlm.nih.gov/pubmed/22593941

Douillard, J. 2020. "5 Ayurvedic spices to rock your digestive world". https://lifespa.com/five-ayurvedic-spices-digestion

Douillard, J. 2020. "Kitchari: Ayurveda's #1 superfood for cleaning and rejuvenation (+ Recipe)". https://lifespa.com/whats-so-amazing-about-kitchari

Douillard, J., 2019. "Slippery Elm prebiotic tea to restore gut health". https://lifespa.com/tea-psychic-bugs-slippery-elm-prebiotic-tea-formula

Grzanna, R., et. al. 2005. "Ginger--an herbal medicinal product with broad anti-inflammatory actions". J Med Food 8 (2): 125-32. https://doi.org/10.1089/jmf.2005.8.125

Marshall, N. n.d. "Kicharee...Digestion's Best Friend". Mudita Institute & Health Clinic, Australia. https://www.muditainstitute.com/resources/blogs/happy-bellyblogs/kichareedigestion.html

McDonald, D., et. al. 2018. "American gut: An open platform for citizen science microbiome research". *mSystems* 3 (3). https://doi.org/10.1128 mSystems.00031-18

Muller-Lissner, et. al. 2005. "The perceived effect of various foods and beverages on stool consistency". *Eur J Gastroenterol Hepatol* 17 (1): 109-12. https://doi.org/10.1097/00042737-200501000-00020

Perkins, C. 2015. "SIBO Treatment, Diet and Maintenance". Holistic Health. https://www.holistichelp.net/blog/sibo-treatment-diet-and-maintenance

Sánchez-Hervása, M., et al. 2008. "Mycobiota and mycotoxin producing fungi from cocoa beans". International Journal of Food Microbiology 125 (3): 336-40. https://doi.org/10.1016/j.ijfoodmicro.2008.04.021

The Barral Institute. n.d. "Discover Visceral Manipulation". https://discovervm.com

University of California, San Diego. 2018. "Big data from world's largest citizen science microbiome project serves food for thought. How factors such as diet, antibiotics and mental health status can influence the microbial and molecular makeup of your gut". https://www.sciencedaily.com/releases/2018/05/180515092931.htm Index

# INDEX

# ABOUT THE AUTHOR

Ada J. Peters, is a German-born Australian author. What started as a project to understand and improve her own health evolved into comprehensive research and a commitment to providing others with insightful information about the gut and beyond. She faced multiple health issues related to the gastrointestinal tract for decades and knows all too well that there is no one-size-fits-all solution. Her mantra is not to give up, to continue to educate yourself and take one step at a time as each step brings you closer to better health. When she's not cooking and researching, she's on a hike or splashing in the ocean.